SOME FOODS FOOL YOU . . .

DID YOU KNOW

> . . . not all egg substitutes are low in cholesterol?

> . . . beef franks have less cholesterol than chicken franks?

> . . . a cheeseburger at McDonald's is lower in both calories and cholesterol than a fish sandwich?

THE QUICK AND EASY CHOLESTEROL & CALORIE COUNTER

COMPILED BY
LYNN SONBERG

AVON BOOKS ◆ NEW YORK

Before beginning any diet, the reader should consult his or her physician and should specifically discuss the intended diet with the physician.

AVON BOOKS
A division of
The Hearst Corporation
105 Madison Avenue
New York, New York 10016

Copyright © 1988 by Lynn Sonberg
Published by arrangement with Lynn Sonberg Book Services
Library of Congress Catalog Card Number: 88-91529
ISBN: 0-380-75573-4

First Avon Books Printing: October 1988

AVON TRADEMARK REG. U.S. PAT. OFF. AND IN OTHER COUNTRIES, MARCA REGISTRADA, HECHO EN U.S.A.

Printed in the U.S.A.

K-R   10   9   8   7   6   5   4   3   2   1

Acknowledgments

Most of the cholesterol and calorie information for brand-name foods was supplied by the manufacturers, in response to our requests. We are thankful for their cooperation. We are also grateful to Nutrient Research Group of the United States Department of Agriculture for supplying especially difficult to find cholesterol data. The U.S. Department of Agriculture's HANDBOOK NO.8 was another primary source of the nutrition information used in this book. Special thanks are also owed to Matthew Ostrowski for his invaluable help in researching this book.

TABLE OF CONTENTS

INTRODUCTION

WHY ALL THE FUSS ABOUT CHOLESTEROL?

More than ever before, Americans are aware that the foods they eat affect their health. For example, you probably know that too much dietary cholesterol may increase the risk of heart disease. But most people, especially those without special health problems, think the cholesterol issue simply doesn't apply to them. If you are basically healthy, do you really need to be concerned about your cholesterol intake? Unfortunately, the answer is yes. More than half a million people die of heart disease in this country each year. If you, like most Americans, consume a diet high in cholesterol and saturated fat, you have a fifty-fifty chance of dying from some form of heart disease.

These statistics paint a gloomy picture to be sure, but they are by no means inevitable. By giving you the specific nutrition information you need to make healthier, low-cholesterol food choices, this book can help you improve the odds.

Of course, diet is not the sole determining factor in heart disease. Heredity, cigarette smoking, lack of exercise, and certain ailments such as high blood pressure and diabetes also increase your risks. Still, experts today generally agree that the amount of cholesterol in your blood (called your serum cholesterol level) is the single most reliable predictor of whether or not you will develop atherosclerosis, the most common form of heart disease. The bottom line is: you can lower your serum cholesterol level through diet. If you reduce your cholesterol level by only 10

1

percent, for example, studies show that your heart attack risk will drop a full 20 percent! On a national scale, this modest reduction could save 100,000 lives a year. Needless to say, greater reductions would yield even greater benefits.

Before we explain how to use this book to help you make heart-healthy food choices, it may help to understand more about cholesterol's role in health and disease.

WHAT IS CHOLESTEROL?

Cholesterol is a waxy, fatlike substance used by the body for vital metabolic processes including cell growth and the manufacture of hormones and certain vitamins. It occurs in foods of animal origin like meat, fish, eggs, and dairy products, and is also produced by the human body. While cholesterol is essential to normal functioning, the liver produces 1,000 milligrams each day, more than enough for the body's needs. High blood levels of cholesterol most often result from high dietary intake. Research shows that consumption of up to 100 mg of dietary cholesterol each day will not affect blood levels. But the average consumption in this country is 450–600 mg daily! This excess cholesterol can be deposited on artery walls, leading to atherosclerosis, the most common form of heart disease. When an artery feeding the heart becomes so blocked that blood cannot pass, a heart attack occurs.

THE "GOOD" AND "BAD" CHOLESTEROL

Cholesterol does not circulate directly in the blood, but is first "packaged" in envelopes called lipoproteins. High-density lipoproteins, or HDLs, carry cholesterol back to the liver where it is excreted in the bile. In other words, HDLs (the "good" cholesterol) actually help to lower serum levels. In contrast, low-density lipoproteins, or LDLs carry cholesterol throughout the body, supplying it to cells as needed, but also depositing some of the excess on artery walls. A high ratio of HDL cholesterol to LDL cholesterol helps protect against heart disease.

WHAT SHOULD YOUR CHOLESTEROL LEVEL BE?

The standard laboratory test measures how much cholesterol by weight is contained in a given volume of blood. The standard unit of weight used is the milligram (mg) and the standard unit of volume used is the deciliter (dl). Frequently you will find cholesterol levels given simply as 200 mg or simply 200. This is a shorthand way of saying 200 milligrams per deciliter of blood.

According to the latest government guidelines, issued in October 1987 by the National Cholesterol Education Program, all Americans should have their cholesterol levels tested beginning at age twenty. If you are thirty years of age or older, a cholesterol level of 200 milligrams per deciliter of blood is considered desirable. When the level tops 200, the risk of heart attack climbs sharply. (Younger people should aim for a count of 180 mg or less.) LDL-cholesterol (the "bad" kind) should be kept below 130 milligrams per deciliter. While a desirable level for HDL (the "good") cholesterol has not been set, the new guidelines say that levels below 35 milligrams per deciliter are a major risk factor.

Early testing is important for several reasons. First, it establishes a baseline measurement to help your physician assess changes in your blood chemistry as you grow older. Obviously, if your cholesterol level is already above the recommended guidelines at age twenty, you will want to make changes in your diet before the problem worsens. Early testing can also reveal elevated LDL-levels due to a genetic defect that predisposes carriers to heart attacks before middle age. For the estimated 400,000 Americans who have this genetic defect, early testing, followed by dietary and/or drug therapy, can literally be lifesaving.

It is important to realize that some health scientists believe that the government recommendations regarding "desirable" cholesterol levels still fall short of the ideal.

A major research program involving more than 350,000 men over an eight-year period, for example, showed that the risk of heart attack begins to rise once cholesterol levels exceed 150 mg/dl. While it is certainly true that the "zone of accelerated risk" is above 200, individuals with cholesterol levels between 182 and 202 were still 29 percent more likely to die prematurely from heart disease than men with levels below 180.

In short, many health scientists believe that the optimum cholesterol level for adults thirty years and older should be 180 mg/dl or even lower. In their view, the government guidelines should be viewed as a minimum standard.

This example of divided opinion among health authorities is not unusual. The science of nutrition is a new and constantly evolving field. It takes many years of carefully designed research studies before scientists have enough evidence to make recommendations about what we should and should not eat. So while today we know a great deal more about how diet contributes to—or helps protect against—heart disease than we used to, chances are that "official" recommendations will continue to evolve as new scientific evidence comes to light.

Here is a summary of the 1987 government guidelines for identifying and treating individuals with elevated cholesterol levels:

- **DESIRABLE** blood cholesterol level: less than 200 mg/dl. LDL cholesterol less than 130.

Recommendation: Recheck every five years.

- **BORDERLINE HIGH** blood cholesterol level: 200–239 mg/dl. LDL cholesterol is 130–159.

Recommendation: Follow STEP 1 DIET: Restrict total fat intake to less than 30 percent of calories, saturated fat to less than 10 percent of calories, and cholesterol intake to less than 300 milligrams per day. Recheck cholesterol level annually.

- **BORDERLINE HIGH WITH RISK FACTORS** blood cholesterol level: 200–239 mg/dl, LDL cholesterol is 130–159, and individual has one or more risk factors, e.g., family history of premature coronary heart disease, cigarette smoking, high blood pressure, low level of HDL-cholesterol, diabetes, history of stroke or blockage of blood vessels in other body parts, severe obesity. Women should consider themselves in this category if two of these risk factors are present. Men should consider themselves in this category if one risk factor is present. Anyone who already has coronary heart disease is in this category.

Recommendation: Additional test for LDL-cholesterol level, followed by STEP 1 DIET (see above) under medical supervision with three additional tests to monitor blood cholesterol level, taken over three months. If this diet fails to achieve desired goals, STEP 2 DIET is recommended. This diet further reduces saturated fat to less than 7 percent of total calories and cholesterol intake to less than 200 mg per day. If six months of this diet fails, drug treatment may be recommended, in addition to the STEP 2 DIET.

———————————

- **HIGH RISK** blood cholesterol level: 240 or higher. LDL-cholesterol is 160 or higher.

Recommendation: Same as borderline high with risk factors, above.

———————————

HEALTHY LOW-CHOLESTEROL EATING

Dietary changes can dramatically alter your blood cholesterol levels. Keeping your intake of cholesterol low is important, to be sure, and you should use this guide to keep track of the amount of cholesterol you are consuming. But your overall diet must be heart-healthy as well. It is especially important, for example, to limit your intake of saturated fat, which tends to raise cholesterol levels.

Here are some guidelines for healthy eating recommended by major government and health organizations.*

1. Limit consumption of cholesterol, saturated fat, and overall fat.

Cholesterol should be limited to less than 300 mg per day. If your cholesterol level remains elevated, cholesterol intake should be further reduced to 200 mg a day.

All types of fat and oil, especially saturated fat, should also be limited. Foods high in saturated fat and cholesterol include meats (especially red meats) butter, cheese, eggs, and whole milk products. Saturated fat is also "hidden" in many processed foods such as bakery goods, cereals, nondairy creamers and other unlikely sources. Get in the habit of checking ingredients lists for coconut oil, palm oil, vegetable shortening, and lard, which are the most highly saturated fats. Hydrogenated and partially hydrogenated vegetable oils should also be avoided.

You should get no more than 30 percent of your calories from fat, and no more than one-third of this amount from saturated fat. Monounsaturated fats such as olive oil and peanut oil as well as polyunsaturated fats tend to lower cholesterol levels. But even these fats, which are beneficial, should only be eaten in very small amounts.

2. Increase your consumption of fish.

There is one type of fat you should eat more of: Omega-3 fatty acid, which is found in fish and shellfish. Try to eat a small portion of fish at least two or three times a week. Fatty fish such as salmon, bluefish, sardines, mackerel,

---

*The recommendations in this book are based on the findings of an expert panel convened by the National Cholesterol Education Program, sponsored by the National Heart Lung and Blood Institute in cooperation with more than twenty major medical associations (1987); the information on healthy eating is also based on guidelines from the American Heart Association (1986), the National Cancer Institute (1984), the National Academy of Sciences National Research Council (1980), and the Surgeon General's "Report on Preventive Medicine" (1980).

and swordfish are the richest sources of Omega-3 but even shellfish and mollusks contain significant amounts of this substance, which is thought to lower cholesterol levels. Shrimp, oysters, lobster, and scallops can all be eaten (in moderate amounts) on a heart-healthy diet.

3. Increase consumption of complex carbohydrates and dietary fiber, especially soluble fiber.

If you are like most Americans, you only consume 15 grams of dietary fiber daily, instead of the recommended 30 to 40 grams. Similarly, you probably get around 28 percent of your total calories from complex carbohydrates instead of the recommended 50 percent or more.

Research has shown that soluble fiber, which is found in beans, oat bran, carrots, and fruits, can help to lower cholesterol levels. Although research clearly shows the benefits of consuming substantial amounts of foods rich in soluble fiber, no one knows exactly why the cholesterol-lowering effect takes place. Some scientists believe that gums and pectins, which are types of soluble fiber, coat the intestines, cutting down on the amount of fat and cholesterol absorbed during digestion. According to another theory, this type of fiber binds with bile acids (which are made from cholesterol) before being excreted from the body, taking excess cholesterol with it.

Remember, although the more familiar *insoluble* fiber found in bran and whole grains has many benefits (including reduced risk for certain types of cancer), only *soluble* fiber helps to lower cholesterol levels.

4. Increase protein intake from vegetable sources.

Try to get used to smaller portions of meat and poultry, using them almost as a condiment. Rely instead on main dishes based on whole grains, legumes (dried peas and beans), vegetables, and soy products. If you can get used to this way of eating, you will automatically be consuming less cholesterol and saturated fat, and at the same time increasing your intake of fiber and complex carbohydrates.

Recent studies show that cruciferous vegetables (such as broccoli, cabbage, brussels sprouts, and cauliflower), as well as vegetables rich in vitamins A and D, may have anticancer properties. Try to increase your consumption of these vegetables.

5. Decrease consumption of salt and refined sugar.

6. Limit consumption of salt-cured, smoked, and pickled foods.

ANSWERING YOUR QUESTIONS ABOUT CHOLESTEROL

The basic purpose of this guide is to enable you to keep track of how much cholesterol you are consuming. While this sounds simple enough, unfortunately the cholesterol count of a given food does not always tell the whole story. It may be fairly low in cholesterol and still be "bad" for you, or fairly high in cholesterol and still be "good" for you. For example, deep-fried shrimp contain less cholesterol than plain shrimp, yet it hardly follows that the fried version is better for you. The reason is simply that the fried version contains less shrimp and more breading (and only the shrimp contain cholesterol).

In this section we'll try to answer some of the questions you may have about interpreting the data in this book, as well as questions about certain foods and their role in an overall heart-healthy diet.

Q: I have a tremendous sweet tooth and am especially fond of chocolate. I see that Hostess Chocolate Cupcakes and Nestlé chocolate bars have hardly any cholesterol. Does this mean I can indulge my sweet tooth without worrying about increasing my risk of heart disease?

A: Unfortunately, no. Even though these products are low in cholesterol, they are high in saturated fat and sugar. Too much saturated fat in your diet will tend to elevate cholesterol levels, even if your cholesterol consumption remains within the recommended guidelines. In fact, some scientists believe that keeping your saturated fat intake low is even more important than restricting cholesterol consumption. The role of sugar consumption in heart disease is not firmly established, but some research indicates that diets high in sugar may be associated with increases in cholesterol and triglyceride levels. (Elevated triglyceride levels in the blood are associated with heart-disease risk.) This may be especially true for some 20 million Americans with a genetic tendency to have high triglyceride levels when consuming a high sugar diet.

Q: Since your listing shows that Wise Potato Chips and Fritos Corn Chips have no cholesterol, I presume I can munch away without worrying about heart disease. Right? I know these foods are fattening, but luckily I don't have to worry about my weight.

A: Wrong. Again the culprit is saturated fat, which should be avoided as much as possible if you are interested in following a heart-healthy diet. Many foods high in cholesterol, such as fatty red meats and whole dairy products, are also high in saturated fat. But saturated fat is often "hidden" in processed foods that contain no cholesterol at all. Often manufacturers will try to trick you into thinking that their products are heart-healthy by saying "no cholesterol" or "made only with vegetable oil." But if the vegetable oil used is saturated or partially hydrogenated, it will have a negative effect on your cholesterol level. To learn whether your favorite convenience foods contain undesirable oils, get into the habit of reading the ingredients list on food labels before you buy. Wise Potato Chips, for example, lists partially hydrogenated vegetable oil, while Fritos lists several oils, including partially hydrogenated sunflower oil. You should also avoid coconut oil, palm kernel oil, and cottonseed oil, which are highly saturated.

Q: I'm confused. I remember reading that shrimp, lobster, and oysters are very high in cholesterol and should be avoided on a cholesterol-restricted diet. Yet the guidelines for healthy eating in this book say that people should eat more fish—including shellfish. Why has shellfish suddenly become healthy?

A: The situation is indeed confusing. To start with, old methods of measuring cholesterol in shellfish were simply inaccurate. Because they could not distinguish cholesterol from other sterol compounds, these methods tended to overstate the actual amount of cholesterol in these foods. Even today, many of the cholesterol counts you may see for shellfish do not reflect the new, more accurate methodology. To add to the confusion, however, even according to the new methodology, the amount of cholesterol in shrimp and lobster, for example, is still higher than what is contained in a well-marbled steak! The reasons these foods are nonetheless heart-healthy have to do with their Omega-3 content (which lowers cholesterol levels) and the fact that, unlike red meat, they contain almost no saturated fat. The same is true for finfish, like salmon, bluefish, or striped bass. Even though their cholesterol content is moderately high, their high Omega-3 content and low saturated fat content make them extremely desirable foods.

Q: I don't understand why the listings in this book show that there is usually more cholesterol in cooked food than in the same amount of the same food when it is raw.

A: The reason isn't difficult to understand once you realize that foods lose water and shrink as they cook. A raw 3½ ounce piece of beef round contains 139 calories and 58 mg of cholesterol; a roasted piece the same size contains 194 calories and 82 mg cholesterol. Because it gives up moisture when it cooks, the raw piece of meat will weigh less after it is roasted than before. In other words, 3½ ounces raw vs. cooked are not really equivalent since the raw version contains more moisture, and the cooked version is "denser." In other words, to end up with 3½ ounces cooked, you have to start with a considerably larger piece of meat in the first place. With this in mind, it begins to make sense that the cooked portion of beef contains substantially more calories and cholesterol.

Q: If what you say is true, how come 3½ ounces of roasted duck contains *fewer* calories than the same amount raw?

A: Duck contains a great deal of fat, which melts away during roasting. In the case of extremely fatty meats such as duck, the decrease in calories due to fat loss is *greater than* the calorie increase due to moisture loss.

HOW TO USE THIS BOOK

In order to look up the cholesterol and calorie content of your favorite foods:

1. Turn to the Table of Contents on pages vii–viii and locate the category of the food you are looking up. We've tried to avoid large, sweeping categories like *Desserts* or *Dairy Products* or *Flour Foods*. So if you are looking up "Mrs. Smith's Apple Pie," you will find it in the *Pie* category; if you are looking for Dannon Strawberry Yogurt, you will find it in the *Yogurt* category; if you are looking for Stouffer's Lean Cuisine Glazed Chicken with Vegetable Rice, you will find it listed within the *Entrees* category; and if you are looking for Aunt Jemima Blueberry Pancakes, you will find it listed in the *Pancakes and Waffles* category.
2. Once you have located the category you want in the Table of Contents, turn to the page where the listings begin. The product you are looking up will be listed alphabetically within that category.
3. Each listing gives the name of the product, either by brand name or generically. This is followed by three columns of information. The first column gives the serving size; the second column gives the calorie count for that serving size; and the third column gives the cholesterol count in milligrams for that serving size.

Remember, even if you have no special health problems, health authorities believe that you should limit your cholesterol intake to less than 300 milligrams daily.

Before making any major change in your diet, always consult your physician.

CHOLESTEROL AND
CALORIE COUNTER

ABBREVIATIONS AND SYMBOLS

fl oz	fluid ounce
mg	milligram
na	data not available
oz	ounce
pc	piece
tbsp	tablespoon
tsp	teaspoon
Tr	trace amount
<	less than

All foods are ready to eat or prepared according to package instructions unless otherwise specified.

Product	Measure/ Quantity	Calories	Cholesterol (mg)
	BEEF		
Brain, fried	3½ oz	196	1995
Breakfast strips	2 strips	102	27
Breakfast Strips (Oscar Mayer)	2 strips	80	22
Brisket, braised	3½ oz	241	93
Brisket, flat half, braised	3½ oz	263	91
Brisket, point half, braised	3½ oz	212	95
Chuck, arm pot roast, raw	3½ oz	135	60
Chuck, arm pot roast, braised	3½ oz	231	101
Chuck, blade roast, braised	3½ oz	270	106
Corned beef, cooked	3½ oz	372	93
Flank steak, braised	3½ oz	244	71
Flank steak, broiled	3½ oz	243	70
Hamburger, extra lean, baked, medium	3½ oz	250	82
Hamburger, extra lean, baked, well done	3½ oz	274	107
Hamburger, extra lean, broiled, medium	3½ oz	256	84
Hamburger, extra lean, fried, medium	3½ oz	255	81
Hamburger, extra lean, raw	3½ oz	234	69
Hamburger, lean, baked, medium	3½ oz	268	78
Hamburger, lean, broiled, medium	3½ oz	272	87
Hamburger, lean, broiled, well done	3½ oz	280	101
Hamburger, lean, fried, medium	3½ oz	275	84
Hamburger, regular, raw	3½ oz	310	85
Hamburger, regular, baked, medium	3½ oz	287	87

Product	Measure/ Quantity	Calories	Cholesterol (mg)
BEEF			
Hamburger, regular, broiled, medium	3½ oz	289	90
Hamburger, regular, fried, medium	3½ oz	306	89
Hamburger, regular, fried, well-done	3½ oz	286	98
Kidneys, simmered	3½ oz	144	387
Liver, fried	3½ oz	217	482
Porterhouse steak, broiled	3½ oz	218	80
Pot roast, braised	3½ oz	231	101
Rib eye, broiled	3½ oz	223	79
Rib, large end, broiled	3½ oz	233	82
Rib, large end, roasted	3½ oz	244	81
Rib, small end, broiled	3½ oz	221	80
Rib, small end, roasted	3½ oz	236	80
Round, raw	3½ oz	139	58
Round, broiled	3½ oz	194	82
Round, bottom, braised	3½ oz	222	96
Round, eye, roasted	3½ oz	183	69
Round, tip, roasted	3½ oz	190	81
Round, top, broiled	3½ oz	191	84
Short ribs, braised	3½ oz	295	93
Sizzlean, Beef (Swift)	2 strips	50	15
Sweetbreads, calf	3½ oz	96	462
T-Bone steak, raw	3½ oz	159	60
T-Bone steak, broiled	3½ oz	214	80
Tenderloin, broiled	3½ oz	204	84
Tenderloin, roasted	3½ oz	219	86
Tongue, simmered	3½ oz	283	107
Top loin, broiled	3½ oz	203	76
Tripe, raw	3½ oz	98	95
Wedge-bone sirloin, raw	3½ oz	136	61
Wedge-bone sirloin, broiled	3½ oz	208	89

Product	Measure/ Quantity	Calories	Cholesterol (mg)
BEVERAGES			

BEER

Product	Measure/ Quantity	Calories	Cholesterol (mg)
Ale	12 fl oz	147	0
Beer	12 fl oz	156	0
Beer, light	12 fl oz	100	0

CARBONATED DRINKS

Product	Measure/ Quantity	Calories	Cholesterol (mg)
Bitter Lemon	12 fl oz	192	0
Club Soda/Seltzer	12 fl oz	0	0
Coca-Cola	12 fl oz	144	0
Cream Soda	12 fl oz	156	0
Diet Coke	12 fl oz	1	0
Diet Pepsi	12 fl oz	1	0
Diet 7-Up	12 fl oz	4	0
Fresca	12 fl oz	4	0
Ginger Ale	12 fl oz	113	0
Grape Soda	12 fl oz	179	0
Mountain Dew	12 fl oz	171	0
Orange Soda	12 fl oz	179	0
Perrier	12 fl oz	0	0
Pepsi-Cola	12 fl oz	156	0
RC Cola	12 fl oz	156	0
Root Beer	12 fl oz	163	0
7-Up	12 fl oz	144	0
Sprite	12 fl oz	144	0
Tab	12 fl oz	1	0
Vernor's	12 fl oz	139	0

COFFEE

Product	Measure/ Quantity	Calories	Cholesterol (mg)
Brewed	6 fl oz	3	0
Instant, flavored			
Almond Mocha	6 fl oz	64	na
Cafe Amaretto	6 fl oz	51	Tr
Cafe Vienna	6 fl oz	64	Tr
Orange Cappucino	6 fl oz	64	0

DISTILLED LIQUORS (ALL VARIETIES)

Product	Measure/ Quantity	Calories	Cholesterol (mg)
80 proof	1 fl oz	65	0
90 proof	1 fl oz	74	0
100 proof	1 fl oz	83	0

Product	Measure/ Quantity	Calories	Cholesterol (mg)

BEVERAGES

JUICES: FRUIT/VEGETABLE

Product	Measure/ Quantity	Calories	Cholesterol (mg)
Apple, bottled	8 fl oz	116	0
Apple, frozen	8 fl oz	111	0
Carrot, fresh	8 fl oz	96	0
Grape, bottled	8 fl oz	155	0
Grape, frozen	8 fl oz	128	0
Grapefruit, frozen	8 fl oz	102	0
Orange, canned	8 fl oz	104	0
Orange, frozen	8 fl oz	112	0
Pineapple, canned	8 fl oz	137	0
Prune, bottled	8 fl oz	181	0
Tomato	8 fl oz	41	0

PUNCHES, JUICE DRINKS

Product	Measure/ Quantity	Calories	Cholesterol (mg)
Cranberry Juice Cocktail (Ocean Spray)	8 fl oz	147	0
Five Alive Fruit Punch	8 fl oz	87	0
Gatorade	8 fl oz	39	0
Hawaiian Punch	8 fl oz	89	0
Lemonade, frozen	8 fl oz	96	0
Tang	6 fl oz	89	0

TEA

Product	Measure/ Quantity	Calories	Cholesterol (mg)
Brewed	6 fl oz	0	0
Herbal	6 fl oz	0	0
Iced, instant	6 fl oz	2	0

WINE

Product	Measure/ Quantity	Calories	Cholesterol (mg)
Champagne	4 oz	84	0
Red	3½ oz	76	0
Sauterne	3½ oz	84	0
Sherry	2 fl oz	84	0
White	3½ oz	80	0

BREAD, MUFFINS, AND ROLLS

BAGELS

Product	Measure/ Quantity	Calories	Cholesterol (mg)
Egg (Lender's)	1 bagel	150	<5
Onion (Lender's)	1 bagel	160	<5
White, plain	1 bagel	163	0

Product	Measure/ Quantity	Calories	Cholesterol (mg)

BREAD, MUFFINS, AND ROLLS

Product	Measure/ Quantity	Calories	Cholesterol (mg)
Biscuits (Wonder)	2 biscuits	200	<5
Black Bread (Levy's)	2 slices	140	0
Bran'nola Country Oat	2 slices	220	<5
Bran'nola Hearty White	2 slices	210	<5
Bran'nola Old Style White	2 slices	170	0
Breadcrumbs (Progresso)	½ cup	173	0
Brown, canned	2,½" slices	160	na
Cornbread, Southern style	1 pc	172	58
Cracked Wheat (Pepperidge Farm)	2 slices	140	<5
Cracked Wheat (Wonder)	2 slices	150	<5
French Bread	2 oz	84	0
French Style (Francisco)	2 oz	160	0
Fresh Horizons Wheat	2 slices	100	0
Hollywood, Dark	2 slices	136	Tr
Hollywood, Light	2 slices	136	Tr
Honey Wheat Berry (Arnold)	2 slices	180	<5
Honey Wheat Berry (Pepperidge Farm)	2 slices	140	0
Italian	2 oz	84	0
Low Sodium (Wonder)	2 slices	140	<5
MUFFINS			
Apple Cinnamon Spice (Sara Lee)	1 muffin	220	0
Blueberry (Morton)	1 muffin	125	9
Blueberry (Sara Lee)	1 muffin	200	0
Bran (Arnold Branola)	1 muffin	160	0
Corn (Morton)	1 muffin	129	14
English (Thomas')	1 muffin	133	<5
Homemade	1 muffin	120	21
Pita (Sahara)	1 loaf	80	0
Raisin (Arnold Tea)	2 slices	140	<5
Raisin (Thomas Cinnamon)	2 slices	120	Tr
ROLLS			
Dinner Rolls (Home Pride)	2 rolls	170	<5

Product	Measure/ Quantity	Calories	Cholesterol (mg)
BREAD, MUFFINS, AND ROLLS			
Dinner Rounds (Arnold)	2 rolls	110	<5
Dutch Egg Sandwich Buns	1 roll	130	<5
French (Pepperidge Farm)	½ roll	180	0
Hamburger (Arnold)	1 roll	110	0
Hamburger (Wonder)	1 roll	162	<5
Hot Dog (Arnold)	1 roll	110	0
Hot Dog (Wonder)	1 roll	120	<5
Kaiser (Wonder)	½ roll	230	<5
Pan Rolls (Wonder)	2 rolls	200	<5
Sandwich Rolls (Francisco)	1 roll	160	0
Sandwich Rolls with Poppy Seeds (Arnold)	1 roll	110	<5
Sourdough French Rolls (Francisco)	1 roll	90	0
White (Pipin'Hot)	2 rolls	153	0
Whole Wheat (Pipin'Hot)	2 rolls	155	na
Roman Meal	2 slices	140	<5
RYE BREADS			
Arnold Pumpernickel	2 slices	150	0
Dill Rye (Arnold)	2 slices	150	0
Grossinger's	2 slices	140	0
Grossinger's Pumpernickel	2 slices	140	0
Grossinger's Seeded	2 slices	140	0
Levy's	2 slices	160	0
Levy's Pumpernickel	2 slices	170	0
Melba Thin	2 slices	100	0
Pepperidge Farm	2 slices	170	0
Wonder	2 slices	140	<5
Seven Grain (Home Pride)	2 slices	140	<5
Sour Dough (Di Carlo)	2 slices	140	0

Product	Measure/Quantity	Calories	Cholesterol (mg)

BREAD, MUFFINS, AND ROLLS

Product	Measure/Quantity	Calories	Cholesterol (mg)
Thomas' Protogen Protein Bread	2 slices	93	0
Vienna Style (Francisco)	2 oz	160	0
WHITE BREADS			
Arnold Brick Oven	2 slices	130	<5
Country White (Arnold)	2 slices	190	<5
Fresh Horizons	2 slices	100	0
Hearthstone	2 slices	170	0
Home Pride	2 slices	150	<5
Mrs. Wright's	2 slices	120	<5
Pepperidge Farm	2 slices	150	<5
Wonder	2 slices	140	<5
Wonder w/Buttermilk	2 slices	150	<5
WHOLE WHEAT BREADS			
Arnold Brick Oven	2 slices	160	<5
Fresh and Natural	2 slices	140	0
Home Pride Butter Top	2 slices	150	<5
Home Pride 100%	2 slices	140	<5
Matthew's All Natural	2 slices	180	0
Measure Up	2 slices	80	<5
Pepperidge Farm	2 slices	130	<5
Sprouted Wheat (Arnold)	2 slices	130	<5
Sprouted Wheat (Pepperidge Farm)	2 slices	140	0
Stone Ground (Arnold)	2 slices	110	0
Thomas'	2 slices	112	0
Wonder	2 slices	140	<5
Wheatberry (Home Pride)	2 slices	140	Tr

CAKE

Product	Measure/Quantity	Calories	Cholesterol (mg)
DESSERT CAKES			
Angel food, homemade	1/12 cake	161	0
Angel food, from mix	1/12 cake	140	0
Banana (Morton)	2 1/3 oz	160	9

Product	Measure/ Quantity	Calories	Cholesterol (mg)
CAKE			
Carrot (Duncan Hines)	⅟₁₂ cake	250	<1
Cheesecake (Royal)	⅛ cake	230	5
Chocolate, homemade	⅟₁₂ cake	227	43
Chocolate, from mix	⅟₁₆ cake	250	33
Chocolate (Morton)	2⅓ oz	180	9
Coconut (Morton)	2⅓ oz	170	9
Devil's food	⅟₁₆ cake	235	33
Fruitcake	½ oz	55	7
Fruit loaf (Hostess)	2½ oz slice	400	3
Gingerbread	⅟₁₆ cake	175	Tr
Lemon (Morton)	2⅓ oz	160	9
Pound Cake, Cholesterol Free (Sara Lee)	2 oz	220	0
Sponge cake, homemade	⅟₁₂ cake	195	162
White cake	⅟₁₆ cake	250	1
Yellow cake, homemade	⅟₁₆ cake	275	33
SNACK CAKES			
Big Wheels	1	170	6
Chip Flips	1	330	25
Choco-diles	1	240	22
Crumb Cake (Hostess)	1	130	10
Cupcake, Chocolate (Hostess)	1	170	3
Cupcake, Orange (Hostess)	1	150	13
Dessert Cups (Hostess)	1	60	9
Ding Dongs	1	170	6
Fruit Loaf (Hostess)	1	400	7
Ho-Hos	1	120	13
Hostess-O's	1	240	14
Peanut Putters, Filled	1	360	4
Peanut Putters, Unfilled	1	410	4
Ring Ding	1	160	6
Suzy Q's, Banana	1	240	21
Suzy Q's, Chocolate	1	240	16

Product	Measure/ Quantity	Calories	Cholesterol (mg)

CAKE

Product	Measure/ Quantity	Calories	Cholesterol (mg)
Tiger Tail	1	210	25
Twinkies	1	160	20

CANDY

Product	Measure/ Quantity	Calories	Cholesterol (mg)
Baby Ruth	1 bar	300	0
Butterfinger	1 bar	220	0
Butterscotch morsels	1 oz	150	1
Candy corn	1 oz	56	0
Cracker Jack	1 oz	120	0
Dark Chocolate (Hershey)	1 bar	157	0
Gum drops	1 oz	97	0
Hard candy	6 pc	108	0
Jellybeans	10	66	0
Lifesavers	1 pc	10	0
M&M's, Peanut	1 bag	240	5
M&M's, Plain	1 bag	240	5
Marshmallows (Kraft)	1 pc	25	0
Milk Chocolate (Hershey)	1 bar	160	10
Milk Chocolate (Nestlé)	1 bar	160	5
Milk Chocolate with Almonds (Hershey)	1 bar	160	5
Milk Chocolate with Almonds (Nestlé)	1 bar	150	5
Milky Way	1 bar	270	10
Nestlé Crunch	1 bar	160	6
Peanut Brittle (Planters)	1 oz	123	0
Reese's Peanut Butter Cups	2 pc	240	4
Toffee (Kraft)	1 pc	30	0

CEREALS

COLD CEREALS

Product	Measure/ Quantity	Calories	Cholesterol (mg)
All-Bran (Kellogg)	1 oz	70	0
All-Bran with extra fiber (Kellogg)	1 oz	70	0

Product	Measure/ Quantity	Calories	Cholesterol (mg)
	CEREALS		
Alpha-Bits	1 oz	120	0
Apple Jacks	1 oz	110	0
Bran Buds	1 oz	80	0
Bran Chex	1 oz	96	0
Cap'n Crunch	1 oz	131	0
Cap'n Crunch's Crunchberries	1 oz	130	0
Cheerios	1 oz	120	0
Cocoa Crispies	1 oz	120	0
Cocoa Pebbles	1 oz	120	0
Cocoa Puffs	1 oz	120	0
Cookie Crisp	1 oz	190	0
Corn Bran	1 oz	120	0
Corn Chex	1 oz	120	0
Corn Pops	1 oz	120	0
Cracklin' Oat Bran	1 oz	113	0
Crispix	1 oz	110	0
Crispy Wheats 'n Raisins	1 oz	120	0
C.W. Post	1 oz	131	0
Fiber One	1 oz	60	0
Froot Loops	1 oz	190	0
Frosted Flakes	1 oz	110	0
Frosted Mini-Wheats	1 oz	110	0
Fruit & Fibre	1 oz	90	0
Fruity Pebbles	1 oz	120	0
Golden Grahams	1 oz	120	0
Grape-Nuts	1 oz	120	0
Grape-Nuts Flakes	1 oz	107	0
Health Valley Sprouts 7	1 oz	110	0
Heartland	1 oz	128	0
Honeycomb	1 oz	120	0
Honey Nut Cheerios	1 oz	120	0
Honey Nut Crunch Raisin Bran	1 oz	90	0
Honey Smacks	1 oz	120	0
Kellogg's 40% Bran Flakes	1 oz	90	0

Product	Measure/ Quantity	Calories	Cholesterol (mg)

CEREALS

Product	Measure/ Quantity	Calories	Cholesterol (mg)
Kellogg's Corn Flakes	1 oz	120	0
Kellogg's Raisin Bran	1 oz	120	0
Kix	1 oz	120	0
Life	1 oz	120	0
Lucky Charms	1 oz	120	0
Marshmallow Krispies	1 oz	150	0
Nabisco Shredded Wheat	1 biscuit	100	0
Nabisco 100% Bran	1 oz	70	0
Nature Valley Granola	1 oz	131	0
Nutri-Grain, Corn	1 oz	110	0
Nutri-Grain, Rye	1 oz	107	0
Nutri-Grain, Wheat	1 oz	110	0
Pac-Man	1 oz	110	0
Post 40% Bran Flakes	1 oz	100	0
Post Raisin Bran	1 oz	90	0
Post Toasties Corn Flakes	1 oz	110	0
Product 19	1 oz	110	0
Quaker 100% Natural Cereal	1 oz	114	0
Ralston Purina 40% Bran	1 oz	97	0
Rice Chex	1 oz	120	0
Rice Krispies	1 oz	110	0
Shredded Wheat 'n Bran	1 oz	110	0
Smurf-Berry Crunch	1 oz	120	0
Special K	1 oz	110	0
Super Sugar Crisp	1 oz	111	0
Total	1 oz	120	0
Trix	1 oz	120	0
Wheat Chex	1 oz	110	0
Wheaties	1 oz	104	0

HOT CEREALS

Product	Measure/ Quantity	Calories	Cholesterol (mg)
Buckwheat Groats (Pocono)	1 oz	na	Tr
Cream of Rice	½ cup	63	0
Cream of Wheat, Quick	½ cup	110	0
Farina	½ cup	102	0
Hominy Grits	½ cup	206	0

Product	Measure/ Quantity	Calories	Cholesterol (mg)
CEREALS			
Malt-O-Meal	½ cup	105	0
Maypo	½ cup	100	0
Oatmeal (Quaker)	½ cup	100	0

CHEESE

NATURAL			
Blue	1 oz	100	21
Brick	1 oz	105	27
Brie	1 oz	95	28
Burger Cheese			
(Sargento)	1 oz	106	27
Cajun (Sargento)	1 oz	110	28
Camembert	1 oz	85	20
Caraway	1 oz	107	na
Cheddar	1 oz	114	30
Cheddar, grated	1 cup	455	119
Cheddar, New York			
(Sargento)	1 oz	114	30
Cheshire	1 oz	110	29
Colby	1 oz	112	27
Colby-Jack (Sargento)	1 oz	109	27
Cottage, creamed	½ cup	117	17
Cottage, dry curd	½ cup	62	5
Cottage, low fat, 1% fat	½ cup	82	5
Cream cheese	1 oz	99	31
Cream Cheese with			
Chives (Philadelphia)	1 oz	100	25
Edam	1 oz	101	25
Farmer's Cheese			
(Sargento)	1 oz	102	26
Feta	1 oz	75	25
Fontina	1 oz	110	33
Gorgonzola (Sargento)	1 oz	100	21
Gouda	1 oz	101	32
Gruyère	1 oz	117	31
Havarti (Sargento)	1 oz	118	31

Product	Measure/ Quantity	Calories	Cholesterol (mg)
CHEESE			
Jarlsberg (Sargento)	1 oz	100	16
Liederkrantz	1 oz	85	na
Limburger	1 oz	93	26
Monterey Jack	1 oz	106	30
Mozzarella	1 oz	80	22
Mozzarella, part skim	1 oz	72	16
Mozzarella with Pizza Spices (Sargento)	1 oz	79	15
Muenster	1 oz	104	27
Nacho Cheese (Sargento)	1 oz	106	27
Neufchâtel	1 oz	74	22
Parmesan, grated	1 tbsp	33	4
Parmesan, hard	1 oz	111	19
Parmesan & Romano Grated Blend (Sargento)	1 oz	111	24
Port du Salut	1 oz	100	35
Provolone	1 oz	100	20
Queso Blanco (Sargento)	1 oz	104	27
Queso de Papa (Sargento)	1 oz	114	30
Ricotta, part skim	½ cup	171	38
Ricotta, whole milk	½ cup	216	63
Romano	1 oz	110	29
Roquefort	1 oz	105	26
String Cheese (Sargento)	1 oz	79	15
String Cheese, smoked (Sargento)	1 oz	79	15
Swiss	1 oz	107	26
Swiss, Finland (Sargento)	1 oz	107	26
Tilsit	1 oz	96	29
Tybo (Sargento)	1 oz	98	23
CHEESE FOOD			
American	1 oz	93	18
American (Kraft)	1 oz	90	20
American (Land O Lakes)	1 oz	110	25
American Flavored (Harvest Moon)	1 oz	70	10

Product	Measure/ Quantity	Calories	Cholesterol (mg)
CHEESE			
American Flavored (Light-Line)	1 oz	50	10
American Flavored (Light n' Lively)	1 oz	70	15
American, Imitation (Kraft)	1 oz	90	5
American Spread (Sargento Cracker Snack)	1 oz	106	27
American Spread (Snack Mate)	1 oz	80	20
American Spread with Pimento (Sargento Cracker Snack)	1 oz	106	27
Brick (Sargento Cracker Snack)	1 oz	95	25
Cheddar (Cracker Barrel)	1 oz	90	20
Cheddar, Sharp (Snack Mate)	1 oz	80	20
Cheddar Flavor (Light-Line)	1 oz	50	10
Cheddar Flavored (Light n' Lively)	1 oz	70	15
Cheddar, Imitation (Sargento)	1 oz	85	2
Cheddar Spread (Snack Mate)	1 oz	80	20
Cheese 'n Bacon Spread (Snack Mate)	1 oz	80	20
Cheez Whiz	1 oz	80	15
Colby Flavor (Light-Line)	1 oz	50	10
Gruyère Spread (Laughing Cow)	1 oz	100	18
Hickory Smoked (Wispride)	1 oz	100	20
Hot Pepper (Sargento)	1 oz	106	27

Product	Measure/ Quantity	Calories	Cholesterol (mg)
CHEESE			
Italian Style Grated Cheeses (Sargento)	1 oz	108	26
Jalapeño (Land O Lakes)	1 oz	90	20
Limburger Spread (Mohawk Valley)	1 oz	70	20
Mozzarella, Imitation (Sargento)	1 oz	80	2
Muenster Flavor (Light-Line)	1 oz	50	10
Monterey Jack (Kraft)	1 oz	90	20
Monterey Jack Flavor (Light-Line)	1 oz	50	10
Mozzarella Flavor (Light-Line)	1 oz	50	10
Onion (Land O Lakes)	1 oz	90	15
Pimiento	1 oz	106	23
Port Wine Cheddar (Kraft)	1 oz	90	20
Provolone Spread (Laughing Cow)	1 oz	74	18
Salami Cheese Food (Land O Lakes)	1 oz	100	20
Smoked	1 oz	91	17
Spread (Golden Velvet)	1 oz	80	15
Swiss (Kraft)	1 oz	90	20
Swiss (Sargento Cracker Snack)	1 oz	95	24
Swiss Flavor (Light-Line)	1 oz	50	10
Taco Cheese (Sargento)	1 oz	109	27
Velveeta	1 oz	80	20
CHEESE SAUCE			
Canned, from cheddar	1 oz	50	8
Dry mix	¼ cup	79	13
Homemade	¼ cup	132	54

Product	Measure/ Quantity	Calories	Cholesterol (mg)

CHICKEN

BROILERS AND FRYERS

Product	Measure/ Quantity	Calories	Cholesterol (mg)
Broilers, fryers, w/skin, raw	3½ oz	215	75
Broilers, fryers, w/skin, fried & batter dipped	3½ oz	289	87
Broilers, fryers, w/skin, fried & flour coated	3½ oz	269	90
Broilers, fryers, w/skin, roasted	3½ oz	239	88
Broilers, fryers, w/skin, stewed	3½ oz	219	78
Broilers, fryers, flesh only, raw	3½ oz	119	70
Broilers, fryers, flesh only, fried	3½ oz	219	94
Broilers, fryers, flesh only, roasted	3½ oz	190	89
Broilers, fryers, flesh only, stewed	3½ oz	177	83
Broilers, fryers, skin only, fried, batter dipped	3½ oz	394	74
Broilers, fryers, skin only, fried, flour coated	3½ oz	502	73
Broilers, fryers, dark meat only, raw	3½ oz	125	80
Broilers, fryers, dark meat w/skin, raw	3½ oz	237	81
Broilers, fryers, dark meat only, fried	3½ oz	239	96
Broilers, fryers, dark meat w/skin, fried, batter dipped	3½ oz	298	89
Broilers, fryers, dark meat w/skin, fried, flour coated	3½ oz	285	92

Product	Measure/ Quantity	Calories	Cholesterol (mg)
CHICKEN			
Broilers, fryers, dark meat only, roasted	3½ oz	205	93
Broilers, fryers, dark meat w/skin, roasted	3½ oz	253	91
Broilers, fryers, dark meat only, stewed	3½ oz	192	88
Broilers, fryers, dark meat w/skin, stewed	3½ oz	233	82
Broilers, fryers, light meat only, raw	3½ oz	114	58
Broilers, fryers, light meat w/skin, raw	3½ oz	186	67
Broilers, fryers, light meat only, fried	3½ oz	192	90
Broilers, fryers, light meat w/skin, fried, batter dipped	3½ oz	277	84
Broilers, fryers, light meat w/skin, fried, flour coated	3½ oz	246	87
Broilers, fryers, light meat only, roasted	3½ oz	173	85
Broilers, fryers, light meat w/skin, roasted	3½ oz	222	84
Broilers, fryers, light meat only, stewed	3½ oz	159	77
Broilers, fryers, light meat w/skin, stewed	3½ oz	201	74
CAPONS			
Meat and skin, raw	3½ oz	234	75
Meat and skin, roasted	3½ oz	229	86
PARTS			
Breast, meat only, raw	½ breast	129	68
Breast, meat and skin, raw	½ breast	250	92
Breast, meat only, fried	½ breast	161	78

Product	Measure/ Quantity	Calories	Cholesterol (mg)
CHICKEN			
Breast, meat and skin, fried, batter dipped	½ breast	364	119
Breast, meat and skin, fried, flour coated	½ breast	218	88
Breast, meat only, roasted	½ breast	142	73
Breast, meat and skin, roasted	½ breast	193	83
Drumstick, meat only, raw	1 drumstick	74	48
Drumstick, meat and skin, raw	1 drumstick	117	59
Drumstick, meat only, fried	1 drumstick	82	40
Drumstrick, meat and skin, fried, batter dipped	1 drumstick	193	62
Drumstick, meat and skin, fried, flour coated	1 drumstick	120	44
Drumstick, meat only, roasted	1 drumstick	76	41
Drumstick, meat and skin, roasted	1 drumstick	112	48
Drumstick, meat only, stewed	1 drumstick	78	40
Drumstick, meat and skin, stewed	1 drumstick	116	48
Giblets, fried, flour coated	3½ oz	277	446
Giblets, simmered	3½ oz	157	393
Liver pâté	2 oz	114	na
Liver, simmered	3½ oz	157	631
Neck, raw	1 neck	148	49
Neck, simmered	1 neck	94	27
Thigh, meat only, raw	1 thigh	82	57
Thigh, meat and skin, raw	1 thigh	199	79
Thigh, meat only, fried	1 thigh	113	53

Product	Measure/ Quantity	Calories	Cholesterol (mg)
CHICKEN			
Thigh, meat and skin, fried, batter dipped	1 thigh	238	80
Thigh, meat and skin, fried, flour coated	1 thigh	162	60
Thigh, meat only, roasted	1 thigh	109	49
Thigh, meat and skin, roasted	1 thigh	153	58
Thigh, meat only, stewed	1 thigh	107	49
Thigh, meat and skin, stewed	1 thigh	158	57
Wing, meat only, raw	1 wing	36	17
Wing, meat and skin, raw	1 wing	109	38
Wing, meat only, fried	1 wing	42	17
Wing, meat and skin, fried, batter dipped	1 wing	159	39
Wing, meat and skin, fried, flour coated	1 wing	103	26
Wing, meat only, roasted	1 wing	43	18
Wing, meat and skin, roasted	1 wing	99	29
Wing, meat only, stewed	1 wing	43	18
Wing, meat and skin, stewed	1 wing	100	28
ROASTERS			
Roasters, meat and skin, raw	3½ oz	216	73
Roasters, meat and skin, roasted	3½ oz	223	76
Roasters, meat only, roasted	3½ oz	167	75
Roasters, dark meat only, roasted	3½ oz	178	75
Roasters, light meat only, roasted	3½ oz	153	75

Product	Measure/ Quantity	Calories	Cholesterol (mg)

CHICKEN

CHICKEN PRODUCTS
Canned chicken	3½ oz	165	na
Liver pâté	2 oz	114	na
Spread, canned	3½ oz	192	na

TYSON CHICKEN PRODUCTS
Batter Gold	3½ oz	285	85
Breast Strips	3½ oz	270	43
Buttermilk	3½ oz	285	71
Delecta Delicious	3½ oz	305	82
Heat N Serve	3½ oz	270	74
Honey Stung	3½ oz	260	90
Lightly Breaded	3½ oz	255	94
Ozark Fry	3½ oz	275	58
Ozark Fry Heat N Serve	3½ oz	270	53
Sandwich Mate	3½ oz	315	40
School Lunch Patty	3½ oz	290	33

CHOCOLATE

Chips (Baker's)	1 oz	147	Tr
Chips (Nestlé)	1 oz	150	5
Chips, Dark (Hershey)	1 oz	150	0
Semi-Sweet (Baker's)	1 oz	130	Tr
Sweetened (Hershey's)	1 oz	150	0
Unsweetened (Baker's)	1 oz	140	Tr
Unsweetened (Nestlé-Choco-Bake)	1 oz	170	0

CONDIMENTS

Au jus gravy, canned	¼ cup	10	Tr
Au jus gravy, mix, prepared with water	¼ cup	5	Tr
Barbecue sauce	¼ cup	47	0
Barbecue Sauce (Kraft)	1 tbsp	23	0
Barbecue Sauce, Hickory (Open Pit)	1 tbsp	23	0

Product	Measure/ Quantity	Calories	Cholesterol (mg)
CONDIMENTS			
Bearnaise sauce, dried, prepared with milk and butter	½ cup	350	95
Beef gravy, canned	¼ cup	31	2
Brown gravy, mix, prepared with water	¼ cup	3	Tr
Burger Sauce (Big H)	1 tbsp	65	4
Catsup	1 tbsp	16	0
Cheese sauce, dried, prepared with milk	¼ cup	77	14
Chicken gravy, canned	¼ cup	48	1
Chicken gravy, mix, prepared with water	¼ cup	21	1
Chili sauce	1 tbsp	16	0
Curry sauce, prepared with milk	¼ cup	68	9
Hollandaise, mix, prepared with milk and butter	¼ cup	175	47
Horseradish	1 tbsp	7	0
Horseradish Sauce (Kraft)	1 tbsp	50	5
Mayonnaise (Best)	1 tbsp	100	10
Mayonnaise (Hellman's)	1 tbsp	100	10
Mayonnaise (Kraft)	1 tbsp	100	5
Mayonnaise, imitation	1 tbsp	60	5
Mayonnaise, Imitation (Miracle Whip)	1 tbsp	70	5
Mayonnaise, reduced calorie	1 tbsp	40	5
Mushroom gravy, canned	¼ cup	30	0
Mushroom gravy, mix, prepared with water	¼ cup	18	Tr
Mushroom sauce, dried, prepared with milk	¼ cup	107	9
Mustard (French's)	1 tbsp	16	0
Mustard (Kraft)	1 tbsp	12	0
Mustard, brown	1 tbsp	14	0
Mustard, yellow	1 tbsp	11	0

Product	Measure/ Quantity	Calories	Cholesterol (mg)

CONDIMENTS

Product	Measure/ Quantity	Calories	Cholesterol (mg)
Onion gravy, mix, prepared with water	¼ cup	20	Tr
Picante Sauce (Tostitos)	6 tbsp	40	1
Pickles (Claussen)	1 oz	4	0
Pork gravy, mix, prepared with water	¼ cup	19	1
Relish (Vlasic)	1 tbsp	20	0
Soy sauce	1 tbsp	11	0
Sandwich Spread (Kraft)	1 tbsp	50	5
Stroganoff sauce, dried, prepared with milk and water	¼ cup	70	10
Sweet and sour sauce	¼ cup	131	Tr
Sweet and sour sauce, from mix	¼ packet	55	0
Tabasco sauce	1 tbsp	Tr	Tr
Taco sauce, bottled, hot	1 tbsp	6	0
Taco Seasoning for Meat (Ortega)	1 oz	90	0
Tartar sauce	1 tbsp	70	5
Tartar Sauce (Hellman's)	1 tbsp	70	5
Tartar Sauce (Kraft)	1 tbsp	70	5
Teriyaki sauce, bottled	1 tbsp	8	0
Teriyaki sauce, dried, prepared with water	¼ cup	33	0
Turkey gravy, canned	¼ cup	31	1
Turkey gravy, mix, prepared with water	¼ cup	22	1
White sauce	¼ cup	102	9
Worcestershire sauce	1 tbsp	12	0

COOKIES

Product	Measure/ Quantity	Calories	Cholesterol (mg)
Animal (Barnum's)	6 pc	70	<5
Apple Bars (Nabisco)	1 bar	110	0
Apple Fruit Sticks (Almost Home)	1	70	0

Product	Measure/ Quantity	Calories	Cholesterol (mg)
COOKIES			
Applesauce Raisin (Almost Home)	2	140	5
Arrowroot Biscuit (National)	6	130	10
Blueberry Fruit Sticks (Almost Home)	1	70	0
Brownie, homemade	1	95	17
Butter Flavored Cookies (Nabisco)	6	130	5
Creme Filled (Cameo)	2	130	<5
Cherry Fruit Sticks (Almost Home)	1	70	0
Chocolate Chip (Duncan Hines)	2	110	na
Chocolate Chip (Chips Ahoy)	3	140	5
Chocolate Chip, from frozen dough (Rich's)	1	138	7
Chocolate Grahams (Nabisco)	3	150	<5
Date Nut Roll (Dromedary)	1 oz	80	0
Fig Newtons	2 pc	106	<5
Fudge Chocolate Chip (Almost Home)	2 pc	130	0
Fudge 'n Chocolate Creme Sandwich (Almost Home)	1	140	5
Fudge Marble (Baker's Bonus)	2 pc	140	<5
Gingerbread (from mix)	2″ square	100	5
Gingersnaps (Nabisco)	4 snaps	67	<5
Graham (Honey Maid)	4 pc	120	na
Ladyfingers	4	326	157
Mallomars	2	130	0
Mint Sandwich (Nabisco)	2 pc	150	<5
Oatmeal (Almost Home)	2	130	5
Oatmeal, from frozen dough (Rich's)	1	125	1

Product	Measure/ Quantity	Calories	Cholesterol (mg)

COOKIES

Product	Measure/ Quantity	Calories	Cholesterol (mg)
Oatmeal Raisin (Almost Home)	2	130	5
Oatmeal and Raisin, from frozen dough (Rich's)	1	122	6
Oreos	2 pc	98	<5
Peanut Butter, from frozen dough (Rich's)	1	128	2
Seville (Pepperidge Farm)	2 pc	110	na
Shortbread (Lorna Doone)	3 pc	140	5
Shortcake (Melt Away)	2	150	10
Sugar, from frozen dough (Rich's)	1	118	6
Sugar Wafers (Nabisco)	8 pc	150	0
Vanilla Wafers (Nabisco)	7 pc	131	5

CRACKERS

Product	Measure/ Quantity	Calories	Cholesterol (mg)
Crispbread (Wasa)	1	56	0
Matzoh	1	78	0
Melba toast	2	30	0
Rice cakes	1	37	0
Ritz	9	150	<5
Rye Wafer	3	90	0
Saltine	4	52	0
Sesame (Ak-Mok)	1 oz	117	<5
Soda	6	130	0
Triscuit	6	140	0
Uneeda Biscuit	3	60	0
Waverley Crackers (Nabisco)	4	70	<5
Wheat Thins (Nabisco)	1 oz	144	0

DIET FOODS AND DRINKS

Product	Measure/ Quantity	Calories	Cholesterol (mg)
DIET BARS			
Slender Chocolate	2 bars	270	<1
Slender Vanilla	2 bars	270	<1

Product	Measure/ Quantity	Calories	Cholesterol (mg)

DIET FOODS AND DRINKS

DIET DRINKS

Product	Measure/ Quantity	Calories	Cholesterol (mg)
Fit & Frosty, Chocolate	¾ oz envelope	74	1
Fit & Frosty, Strawberry	¾ oz envelope	74	1
Fit & Frosty, Vanilla	¾ oz envelope	69	Tr
Slender Chocolate Malt, canned	10 fl oz	220	4
Slender Strawberry, canned	10 fl oz	220	5
Slender Vanilla, canned	10 fl oz	220	5
Slender Dutch Chocolate, instant (prep. w/2% lowfat milk)	1 cup	231	20
Slender Vanilla, instant, 1 cup (prep. w/2% lowfat milk)	1 cup	231	21

DINNERS

ARMOUR CLASSIC LITE DINNERS

Product	Measure/ Quantity	Calories	Cholesterol (mg)
Chicken Breast Marsala	11 oz	270	85
Steak Diane	10 oz	290	90

ARMOUR DINNER CLASSICS

Product	Measure/ Quantity	Calories	Cholesterol (mg)
Beef Burgundy	10½ oz	330	100
Beef Stroganoff	11¼ oz	360	90
Boneless Beef Short Ribs	10½ oz	500	100
Cod Almondine	12 oz	350	100
Chicken Fricassee	11¾ oz	330	70
Lasagna	10 oz	380	75
Salisbury Steak	11 oz	480	90
Seafood Newburg	10½ oz	270	90
Sirloin Tips	11 oz	380	105
Stuffed Green Peppers	12 oz	350	55
Swedish Meatballs	11½ oz	500	105
Sweet and Sour Chicken	11 oz	390	95

Product	Measure/ Quantity	Calories	Cholesterol (mg)

DINNERS

Product	Measure/ Quantity	Calories	Cholesterol (mg)
Sweet & Sour Pork	11½ oz	470	90
Teriyaki Chicken	10½ oz	460	95
Teriyaki Steak	10 oz	360	95
Veal Parmigiana	10¾ oz	370	65
BANQUET DINNERS			
Beans & Frankfurters	10 oz	510	34
Chopped Beef	11 oz	420	76
Meat Loaf	11 oz	440	82
Salisbury Steak	11 oz	495	76
Turkey	10½ oz	385	37
Western	11 oz	630	87
BANQUET EXTRA HELPING DINNERS			
Beef	16 oz	865	120
Lasagna	16½ oz	645	38
Salisbury Steak	18 oz	910	171
Salisbury Steak with Mushroom Gravy	18 oz	890	169
Turkey	19 oz	750	63
BANQUET FAMILY FAVORITES DINNERS			
Chicken & Dumplings	10 oz	420	43
Macaroni & Cheese	10 oz	415	28
Noodles & Chicken	10 oz	340	45
Spaghetti & Meatballs	10 oz	290	28
BANQUET PLATTERS			
Beef	10 oz	460	70
Fish	8¾ oz	445	92
Ham	10 oz	400	49
White Meat Fried Chicken	9 oz	430	105
White Meat Hot 'n Spicy Fried Chicken	9 oz	430	105
KRAFT DRY DINNERS			
American Style Spaghetti Dinner	¾ cup	193	0
Egg Noodle & Cheese	¾ cup	280	45
Egg Noodle & Chicken	¾ cup	240	35
Macaroni & Cheese	¾ cup	300	5

Product	Measure/Quantity	Calories	Cholesterol (mg)
DINNERS			
Macaroni & Cheese Deluxe	¾ cup	260	20
Spaghetti & Meat Sauce Dinner	¾ cup	250	10
Spiral Macaroni & Cheese	¾ cup	300	10
Tangy Italian Style Spaghetti Dinner	¾ cup	193	4
MORTON COUNTRY TABLE DINNERS			
Fried Chicken	15 oz	710	98
Salisbury Steak	15 oz	500	58
Sliced Beef	14 oz	510	87
Slicked Turkey	15 oz	520	45
MORTON DINNERS			
Beans and Franks	10¾ oz	530	44
Beef	10 oz	260	66
Beef Enchilada	11 oz	280	18
Boneless Chicken	10 oz	230	48
Fish	9 oz	260	74
Fried Chicken	11 oz	460	84
Ham	10 oz	440	64
Macaroni and Beef	10 oz	260	18
Macaroni & Cheese	11 oz	320	18
Meat Loaf	11 oz	340	61
Mexican Style	11 oz	300	16
Salisbury Steak	11 oz	290	52
Spaghetti and Meatballs	11 oz	360	27
Turkey	11 oz	340	66
Veal Parmigiana	11 oz	250	36
Western Style	11¾ oz	400	52
MORTON KING SIZE DINNERS			
Boneless Chicken	17 oz	530	142
Fried Chicken	17 oz	860	141
Salisbury Steak	19 oz	780	125
Turkey	19 oz	580	75
Veal Parmigiana	20 oz	600	72

	Measure/ Quantity	Calories	Cholesterol (mg)
Product			

DINNERS

PRITIKIN QUICK CUISINE

Product	Measure/Quantity	Calories	Cholesterol (mg)
Bean Enchilada	13 oz	362	9
Cheese Canneloni	13 oz	393	22
Chicken à L'Orange	11 oz	296	55
Chicken Curry	11 oz	306	57
Chicken Enchilada	13 oz	380	28
Chicken Salsa	11 oz	257	55
Cod in Wine Sauce	11 oz	244	71
Mediterranean Pilaf	11½ oz	219	<1
Pasta Bolognese	11 oz	208	22
Sweet and Sour Chicken	11½ oz	328	55
Vegetable Fettucini	12 oz	277	9
Vegetable Lasagna	15 oz	318	9

DIPS

Product	Measure/Quantity	Calories	Cholesterol (mg)
Bacon & Horseradish (Kraft)	1 oz	50	10
Blue Cheese (Breakstone)	1 oz	na	14
Blue Cheese (Kraft)	1 oz	50	15
Buttermilk (Kraft)	1 oz	80	5
Buttermilk & Bacon (Kraft)	1 oz	80	5
Buttermilk & Onion (Kraft)	1 oz	70	5
Clam (Kraft)	1 oz	45	20
Creamy Cucumber (Kraft)	1 oz	50	10
Creamy Onion (Kraft)	1 oz	50	10
Enchilada (Fritos)	1 oz	35	1
French Onion (Kraft)	1 oz	50	10
Garlic (Kraft)	2 tbsp	60	0
Green Onion (Kraft)	2 tbsp	50	0
Guacamole (Kraft)	2 tbsp	50	0
Jalapeño (Fritos)	1 oz	33	1
Jalapeño (Hain)	1 oz	24	0
Jalapeño (Kraft)	2 tbsp	50	0
Onion Bean (Hain)	1 oz	25	0

Product	Measure/ Quantity	Calories	Cholesterol (mg)
DUCK			
Flesh and skin, raw	3½ oz	404	76
Flesh only, roasted	3½ oz	201	89
Flesh and skin, roasted	3½ oz	337	84
EGGS			
CHICKEN EGGS			
Boiled	1 large	79	274
Fried	1 large	83	246
Omelet, plain	1 large egg	95	248
Poached	1 large	79	273
Scrambled, with milk	1 large	95	248
White	1 large	16	0
Yolk	1 large	63	272
OTHER EGGS			
Duck, whole	1	130	619
Goose, whole	1	267	na
Quail, whole	1	14	76
Turkey, whole	1	137	737
Turtle, whole	3–5	115	na
EGG SUBSTITUTES			
Country Morning	¼ cup	87	297
Egg Beaters	¼ cup	25	0
Egg Beaters with Cheez	¼ cup	65	3
Egg Magic	½ envelope	na	15
Eggstra (Tillie Lewis)	1 serving	43	58
Frozen	¼ cup	96	1
Powder	⅓ oz	44	57
Scramblend (Land O Lakes)	¼ cup	143	233
Scramblers (Morningstar Farms)	¼ cup	61	0
Second Nature (Avoset)	3 tbsp	42	0

	Measure/ Quantity	Calories	Cholesterol (mg)
Product			

ENTREES

GENERIC RECIPES

Product	Measure/Quantity	Calories	Cholesterol (mg)
Beef and vegetable stew	1 cup	210	63
Cheese soufflé	4 oz	240	189
Chicken à la king	1 cup	468	186
Chicken and noodles	1 cup	250	96
Chicken chow mein	1 cup	224	77
Chicken fricassee	1 cup	388	96
Chop suey	1 cup	300	64
Crab, deviled	1 cup	451	244
Crab imperial	1 cup	323	308
Creamed chipped beef	½ cup	209	32
Lobster Newburg	1 cup	459	455
Macaroni and cheese	1 cup	430	42
Meatloaf	3½ oz	160	92
Spaghetti with meatballs	1 cup	332	75
Stuffed pepper	1 large	315	56
Welsh rarebit	1 cup	415	71

BANQUET LIGHT & ELEGANT ENTREES

Product	Measure/Quantity	Calories	Cholesterol (mg)
Beef Teriyaki with Rice & Pea Pods	8 oz	240	45
Chicken in Cheese Sauce with Rice & Broccoli	8¾ oz	295	50
Glazed Chicken with Vegetable Rice	8 oz	240	75
Lasagna Florentine	11¼ oz	280	25
Macaroni & Cheese with Bread Crumb Topping	9 oz	300	5
Shrimp Creole with Rice & Peppers	10 oz	220	120
Spaghetti with Meat Sauce	10¼ oz	290	35

CHUN KING DIVIDER PAK CANNED ENTREES

Product	Measure/Quantity	Calories	Cholesterol (mg)
Beef Chow Mein	7 oz	100	15
Beef Pepper Oriental	7 oz	110	15
Chicken Chow Mein	7 oz	110	15
Pork Chow Mein	7 oz	120	25
Shrimp Chow Mein	7 oz	100	30

Product	Measure/ Quantity	Calories	Cholesterol (mg)

ENTREES

CHUN KING STIR-FRY CANNED ENTREES

Product	Measure/ Quantity	Calories	Cholesterol (mg)
Egg Foo Yung	5 oz	140	140
Chow Mein with Beef	6 oz	290	50
Chow Mein with Chicken	6 oz	220	45
Pepper Steak	6 oz	250	50
Sukiyaki	6 oz	260	50

LIPTON POUR-A QUICHE

3-Cheese	4⅓ oz	230	250
Bacon & Onion	4⅓ oz	230	240
Ham	4⅓ oz	230	235
Spinach & Onion	4⅓ oz	220	230

MORTON BOIL-IN-BAG ENTREES

Beef Patty	5 oz	200	35
Chicken à la King	5 oz	150	27
Creamed Chipped Beef	5 oz	160	17
Sliced Beef	5 oz	120	34
Sliced Chicken	5 oz	130	27
Sliced Turkey	5 oz	120	27
Sloppy Joe	5 oz	210	33
Veal Parmigiana	5 oz	130	24

MORTON KING SIZE ENTREES

Fried Chicken	12 oz	640	128
Salisbury Steak	10.3 oz	500	87
Sliced Turkey	12.3 oz	380	78

MORTON FAMILY MEALS

Beef Stew	8 oz	190	50
Beef Patties with Mushroom Gravy	8 oz	300	54
Beef Patties with Onion	8 oz	300	54
Beef, sliced, with Gravy	8 oz	210	71
Macaroni & Cheese	8 oz	260	22
Meat Loaf with Tomato Sauce	8 oz	200	53
Salisbury Steak with Gravy	8 oz	240	55
Turkey Croquettes with Gravy	8 oz	200	38

Product	Measure/ Quantity	Calories	Cholesterol (mg)

ENTREES

Product	Measure/ Quantity	Calories	Cholesterol (mg)
Turkey, sliced, with			
Gravy	8 oz	200	38
Veal Parmigiana	8 oz	300	49
MORTON STEAK HOUSE DINNERS			
Beef Tenderloin	9½ oz	890	134
Chopped Sirloin	9½ oz	760	134
Rib Eye	9 oz	820	134
Sirloin Strip	9½ oz	760	134
MORTON MEAT PIES			
Beef	7 oz	430	29
Chicken	7 oz	415	35
Turkey	7 oz	420	38
MRS. SMITH'S ENTREES			
Beef Cannelloni	8¼ oz	430	90
Cheese & Meat Sauce			
Manicotti	8¼ oz	500	130
Cheese & Spinach			
Manicotti	8¼ oz	505	80
Chicken Cannelloni	8¼ oz	540	80
Chicken Continental	2 crepes	320	65
Chicken Maison	2 crepes	350	70
Ham & Vegetable Crepes	2 crepes	305	70
Mushroom Quiche	9½ oz	595	75
Quiche Florentine	9½ oz	625	70
Quiche Lorraine	9½ oz	720	95
Shrimp Cannelloni	8¼ oz	500	70
Shrimp Crepes	2 crepes	305	105
STOUFFER'S LEAN CUISINE			
Beef & Pork Cannelloni			
with Mornay Sauce	9⅝ oz	270	50
Breast of Chicken			
Marsala with			
Vegetables	8⅛ oz	190	69
Cheese Cannelloni with			
Tomato Sauce	9⅛ oz	270	35
Chicken à l'Orange with			
Almond Rice	8 oz	270	55

Product	Measure/ Quantity	Calories	Cholesterol (mg)

ENTREES

Product	Measure/ Quantity	Calories	Cholesterol (mg)
Chicken & Vegetables with Vermicelli	12¾ oz	270	50
Chicken Cacciatore with Vermicelli	10⅞ oz	280	55
Chicken Chow Mein with Rice	11¼ oz	250	35
Filet of Fish Divan	12⅜ oz	270	95
Filet of Fish Florentine	9 oz	240	90
Filet of Fish Jardiniere with Souffléed Potatoes	11¼ oz	280	110
Glazed Chicken with Vegetable Rice	8½ oz	260	65
Herbed Lamb with Rice	10⅜ oz	280	70
Linguine with Clam Sauce	9⅝ oz	260	35
Meatball Stew	10 oz	250	80
Oriental Beef with Vegetables & Rice	8⅝ oz	270	45
Oriental Scallops & Vegetables with Rice	11 oz	220	20
Salisbury Steak with Italian Style Sauce and Vegetables	9½ oz	270	110
Shrimp & Chicken Cantonese with Noodles	10⅛ oz	270	130
Spaghetti with Beef & Mushroom Sauce	11½ oz	280	30
Stuffed Cabbage with Meat in Tomato Sauce	10¾ oz	220	45
Tuna Lasagna with Spinach Noodles & Vegetables	9¾ oz	280	25
Turkey Dijon	9½ oz	280	70
Veal Lasagna	10¼ oz	280	90
Veal Primavera	9⅛ oz	250	90
Zucchini Lasagna	11 oz	260	25

Product	Measure/ Quantity	Calories	Cholesterol (mg)

ENTREES

SWIFT INTERNATIONAL ENTREES

Product	Measure/ Quantity	Calories	Cholesterol (mg)
Chicken Cordon Bleu	6 oz	370	85
Chicken Kiev	6 oz	400	105
Chicken Lucerne	6 oz	340	50
Chicken Parmigiana	6 oz	360	50
Chicken Romanoff	6 oz	340	55
Chicken Royale	6 oz	340	50

WORTHINGTON MEATLESS ENTREES

Product	Measure/ Quantity	Calories	Cholesterol (mg)
Chicken Style Pot Pie Vegetarian	8 oz	450	0
Chili, Meatless	½ cup	190	0
Lasagna, Meatless	9 oz	280	0
Stew, Vegetarian	9½ oz	240	0

FAST FOOD

ARBY'S
Entrees

Product	Measure/ Quantity	Calories	Cholesterol (mg)
Arby's sub	1 sub	269	58
Bac 'n Cheddar Deluxe Roast Beef	1 sand- wich	561	78
Beef 'n Cheddar	1 sand- wich	490	51
Chicken Breast	1 sand- wich	592	57
Chicken Breast, roasted	1 sand- wich	254	196
Chicken Club	1 sand- wich	621	108
Chicken Salad	1 sand- wich	386	30
French Dip Roast Beef	1 sand- wich	386	55
Hot Ham 'n Cheese	1 sand- wich	353	50
Junior Roast Beef	1 sand- wich	218	20

Product	Measure/ Quantity	Calories	Cholesterol (mg)

FAST FOOD

Product	Measure/ Quantity	Calories	Cholesterol (mg)
King Roast Beef	1 sand-wich	467	49
Roast Beef Deluxe	1 sand-wich	486	59
Super Roast Beef	1 sand-wich	501	40
Turkey Deluxe	1 sand-wich	375	39
Side Orders			
Baked Potato, plain	1	290	0
Baked Potato, Superstuffed, Broccoli & Cheddar	1	541	24
Baked Potato, Superstuffed, Deluxe	1	648	72
Baked Potato, Superstuffed, Mushroom & Cheese	1	506	21
Baked Potato, Superstuffed, Taco	1	619	145
French Fries, regular	1 order	211	2.2
Beverages			
Chocolate Shake	10.6 fl oz	384	32
Jamocha Shake	10.8 fl oz	424	31
Vanilla Shake	8.8 fl oz	295	30
Desserts			
Apple Turnover	1 turn-over	310	0
Blueberry Turnover	1 turn-over	340	0
Cherry Turnover	1 turn-over	320	0
ARTHUR TREACHER'S			
Entrees			
Chicken, Fried	4.8 oz	369	65
Chicken Sandwich	1	413	3

Product	Measure/ Quantity	Calories	Cholesterol (mg)
FAST FOOD			
Fish, Broiled	5 oz	245	na
Fish, Fried	2 pc	355	56
Fish Sandwich	1	440	42
Krunch Pup	1	203	25
Shrimp, fried	4 oz	381	93
Side Orders			
Chips (French Fries)	4 oz	276	3.6
Chowder	1 bowl	112	9
Cole Slaw	1 order	123	7
BURGER KING			
Entrees			
Bacon Double Cheeseburger	1	510	104
Cheeseburger	1	317	48
Chicken Tenders	6 pc	204	47
Double Beef Whopper	1	887	176
Double Beef Whopper with Cheese	1	970	199
Double Cheeseburger	1	478	96
Double Hamburger	1	394	74
Hamburger	1	275	37
Hash Browns	2 oz	162	1.0
Scrambled Egg Platter	1	468	1.5
Specialty Chicken Sandwich	1	688	82
Specialty Ham & Cheese Sandwich	1	471	70
Whaler	1 sandwich	488	84
Whaler with Cheese	1 sandwich	530	95
Whopper	1	626	94
Whopper Jr.	1	322	41
Whopper with Cheese	1	709	117
Whopper Jr. with Cheese	1	364	52

Product	Measure/ Quantity	Calories	Cholesterol (mg)
FAST FOOD			

Side Orders

Product	Measure/ Quantity	Calories	Cholesterol (mg)
French Fries, regular	2½ oz	227	2.4
Onion Rings, regular	2¾ oz	274	Tr
Dessert			
Apple Pie	4½ oz	305	1.5
Breakfast			
Bacon, Egg, & Cheese Croissan'wich	1	355	249
Hash Browns	1 order	162	2
Scrambled Egg Platter	1 order	468	370
DAIRY QUEEN			
Entrees			
Chicken Sandwich	1	670	75
Double Hamburger	1	530	85
Double Hamburger with Cheese	1	650	95
Fish Sandwich	1	400	50
Fish Sandwich with Cheese	1	440	60
Hamburger	1	360	45
Hamburger with Cheese	1	410	50
Super Hot Dog	1	520	80
Super Hot Dog with Cheese	1	580	100
Super Hot Dog with Chili	1	570	100
Triple Hamburger	1	710	135
Triple Hamburger with Cheese	1	820	145
Desserts			
Banana Split	13.5 oz	540	30
Buster Bar	5.25 oz	460	10
Chocolate Malt, regular	14 fl oz	760	50
Chocolate Shake, regular	14 fl oz	710	50

Product	Measure/ Quantity	Calories	Cholesterol (mg)

FAST FOOD

Product	Measure/ Quantity	Calories	Cholesterol (mg)
Chocolate Sundae, regular	6 fl oz	310	20
Dilly Bar	1 bar	210	10
Dipped Chocolate Cone, regular	5.5 oz	340	20
Double Delight	1	490	25
Float	14 fl oz	410	20
Freeze	14 fl oz	500	30
Mr. Misty, regular	11.6 fl oz	250	0
Parfait	10 oz	430	30
Soft Ice Cream Cone, regular	5 oz	240	15
Strawberry Shortcake	11 oz	540	25
DOMINO'S PIZZA			
Cheese	2 slices	400	40
Pepperoni	2 slices	440	60
JACK IN THE BOX			
Entrees			
Bacon Cheeseburger Supreme	1	724	70
Cheeseburger	1	323	42
Chicken Supreme	1	601	60
Club Pita	1 sandwich	284	43
Ham & Swiss Burger	1	638	117
Hamburger	1	276	29
Jumbo Jack	1 burger	485	64
Jumbo Jack with Cheese	1 burger	630	110
Moby Jack	1 sandwich	444	47
Mushroom Burger	1	477	87
Pasta Seafood Salad	1 order	394	48
Sirloin Steak Dinner	1	699	75
Swiss & Bacon Burger	1	643	99
Taco, Regular	1	191	21

Product	Measure/ Quantity	Calories	Cholesterol (mg)
FAST FOOD			
Taco Salad	1 order	377	102
Taco, Super	1	288	37
Side Orders			
Cheese Nachos	1 order	571	55
French Fries, regular	1 order	221	8
Onion Rings	1 order	382	27
Beverages			
Chocolate Shake	10.8 fl oz	330	25
Strawberry Shake	11 fl oz	320	25
Vanilla Shake	10.7 fl oz	320	25
Breakfast			
Apple Turnover	1 pc	410	15
Bacon	2 slices	70	10
Breakfast Jack	1	307	203
Canadian Crescent	1 pc	452	226
Pancake Breakfast with Bacon & Syrup	1 order	630	85
Sausage Crescent	1 pc	584	187
Scrambled Eggs Breakfast	1 order	720	260
Supreme Crescent	1 pc	547	178
KENTUCKY FRIED CHICKEN			
Entrees			
Extra Crispy Drumstick	1	173	65
Extra Crispy Side Breast	1	354	67
Extra Spicy Thigh	1	371	121
Extra Spicy Wing	1	218	63
Kentucky Nuggets	6 pc	276	71
Original Recipe Drumstick	1	147	81
Original Recipe Side Breast	1	276	96
Original Recipe Thigh	1	278	122
Original Recipe Wing	1	181	67

Product	Measure/ Quantity	Calories	Cholesterol (mg)

FAST FOOD

Side Orders

Product	Measure/ Quantity	Calories	Cholesterol (mg)
Biscuit	1	269	na
Cole Slaw	2¾ oz	105	4
Corn on the Cob	5 oz	176	0
Kentucky Fries	1 order	268	2
Mashed Potatoes, plain	½ cup	59	0

LONG JOHN SILVER'S

Entrees

Product	Measure/ Quantity	Calories	Cholesterol (mg)
Batter-Fried Fish	1 pc	202	31
Batter-Fried Shrimp	1 order	711	127
Batter-Fried Shrimp	1 pc	47	17
Breaded Clams	1 order	526	2
Breaded Oyster	1 pc	60	5
Breaded Shrimp Platter	1 order	962	122
Breaded Shrimp	1 order	388	96
Chicken Nuggets Dinner	6 pc	699	25
Chicken Plank Dinner	4 pc	1037	25
Clam Dinner	1 order	955	27
Fish & Chicken	1 order	935	56
Fish & Fries	2 pc	651	75
Fish & More	1 order	978	88
Fish Dinner	3 pc	1180	119
Fish Sandwich Platter	1 order	835	75
Kitchen-Breaded Fish	1 pc	122	25
Kitchen-Breaded Fish Dinner	3 pc	940	101
Ocean Chef Salad	1 order	229	64
Oyster Dinner	1 order	789	55
Scallop Dinner	1 order	747	37
Seafood Platter	1 order	976	95
Seafood Salad	1 order	426	113

Side Orders

Product	Measure/ Quantity	Calories	Cholesterol (mg)
Clam Chowder	1 bowl	128	17
Cole Slaw	1 order	182	12
Corn on the Cob	1 order	176	0

Product	Measure/ Quantity	Calories	Cholesterol (mg)
FAST FOOD			
Fries	1 order	247	13
Hushpuppies	2 pc	145	1
Dessert			
Apple Pie	4 oz	280	10
Cherry Pie	4 oz	294	10
Pumpkin Pie	4 oz	251	35
McDONALD'S			
Entrees			
Big Mac	1	253	83
Cheeseburger	1	318	41
Chicken McNuggets	6 pc	323	62
Filet-O-Fish	1 sand-wich	435	47
Hamburger	1	263	29
McD.L.T.	1 burger	680	101
Quarter Pounder	1	427	81
Quarter Pounder with Cheese	1	525	107
Side Orders			
Fries, regular	1 order	220	9
Beverages			
Chocolate Shake	10.2 fl oz	383	30
Strawberry Shake	10.2 fl oz	362	32
Vanilla Shake	10.2 fl oz	352	31
Desserts			
Apple Pie	3 oz	253	12
Caramel Sundae	5.8 oz	361	31
Cherry Pie	3 oz	260	13
Chocolaty Chip Cookies	1 box	342	18
Hot Fudge Sundae	1	357	27
McDonaldland Cookies	1 box	308	10
Soft Serve Cone	4 oz	189	24
Strawberry Sundae	5.8 oz	320	25

Product	Measure/ Quantity	Calories	Cholesterol (mg)

FAST FOOD

Breakfast

Product	Measure/ Quantity	Calories	Cholesterol (mg)
Biscuit with Bacon, Egg, and Cheese	1 biscuit	483	263
Biscuit with Sausage	1 biscuit	467	48
Biscuit with Sausage & Egg	1 biscuit	585	285
Egg McMuffin	1	340	<1
English Muffin with Butter	1	186	15
Hash Browns	2 oz	144	1.4
Hotcakes with Syrup & Butter	1 order	500	47
Sausage McMuffin	1	427	59
Sausage McMuffin with Egg	1	517	287
Scrambled Eggs	1 order	180	514

ROY ROGERS

Entrees

Product	Measure/ Quantity	Calories	Cholesterol (mg)
Bacon Cheeseburger	1	581	103
Cheeseburger	1	563	95
Chicken Leg	1	117	64
Chicken Thigh	1	282	89
Chicken Wing	1	142	52
Hamburger Sandwich	1	456	73
Roast Beef Sandwich	1	317	55
Roast Beef Sandwich with Cheese	1	424	77
Roast Beef Sandwich, large	1	360	73
Roast Beef Sandwich with Cheese, large	1	467	95
RR Bar Burger	1	611	115

Side Dishes

Product	Measure/ Quantity	Calories	Cholesterol (mg)
Baked Potato, Hot Topped Bacon 'n Cheese	1	397	34

Product	Measure/ Quantity	Calories	Cholesterol (mg)
FAST FOOD			
Baked Potato, Hot Topped Sour Cream 'n Chives	1	408	31
Baked Potato, Hot Topped Taco Beef 'n Cheese	1	463	37
Baked Potato, Hot Topped with Margarine	1	274	0
Biscuit	1	231	0
Cole Slaw	1 order	110	0
French Fries, regular	1 order	268	42
Potato Salad	1 order	107	0
Beverages			
Chocolate Shake	11.25 fl oz	358	37
Hot Chocolate	6 fl oz	123	35
Strawberry Shake	11 fl oz	315	37
Vanilla Shake	10.8 fl oz	306	40
Desserts			
Brownie	1	264	10
Caramel Sundae	5 oz	293	23
Strawberry Shortcake	7.2 oz	447	28
Strawberry Sundae	5 oz	216	23
Breakfast			
Apple Danish	1	249	15
Breakfast Crescent Sandwich	1	401	148
Breakfast Crescent Sandwich with Bacon	1	431	156
Breakfast Crescent Sandwich with Ham	1	557	189
Breakfast Crescent Sandwich with Sausage	1	449	168

Product	Measure/ Quantity	Calories	Cholesterol (mg)
FAST FOOD			
Cheese Danish	1	254	11
Cherry Danish	1	271	11
Egg & Biscuit Platter	1 order	394	284
Egg & Biscuit Platter with Bacon	1 order	435	294
Egg & Biscuit Platter with Ham	1 order	442	304
Egg & Biscuit Platter with Sausage	1 order	550	325
Pancake Platter with Syrup & Butter	1 order	452	53
Pancake Platter with Bacon, Syrup & Butter	1 order	493	63
Pancake Platter with Ham, Syrup, & Butter	1 order	506	73
Pancake Platter with Sausage, Syrup, & Butter	1 order	608	94
WENDY'S			
Entrees			
Bacon Cheeseburger	1	460	65
Chicken Sandwich	1	320	59
Chili	8 oz	260	30
Double Cheeseburger	1	630	140
Double Hamburger	1	560	125
Hamburger	1	350	65
Hamburger, Kid's Meal	1	200	20
Triple Cheeseburger	1	1040	225
Side Dishes			
Baked Potato with Bacon & Cheese	1	570	22
Baked Potato with Broccoli & Cheese	1	500	22

Product	Measure/ Quantity	Calories	Cholesterol (mg)

FAST FOOD

Product	Measure/ Quantity	Calories	Cholesterol (mg)
Baked Potato with Cheese	1	590	22
Baked Potato with Chicken à la King	1	350	20
Baked Potato with Chili & Cheese	1	510	22
Baked Potato with Sour Cream & Chives	1	460	15
Baked Potato with Stroganoff & Sour Cream	1	490	43
Baked Potato, plain	1	250	4.8
French Fries, regular	3.5 oz	280	15
Pasta Salad	½ cup	134	0
Breakfast			
Breakfast Sandwich	1	370	200
French Toast	2 slices	400	115
Home Fries	1 order	360	20
Omelet #1, Ham & Cheese	1	250	450
Omelet #2, Ham, Cheese, & mushroom	1	290	355
Omelet #3, Ham, Cheese, Onion, & Green Pepper	1	280	525
Omelet #4, Mushroom, Onion, & Green Pepper	1	210	460
Sausage	1 patty	200	30
Scrambled Eggs	1 order	190	450

Product	Measure/ Quantity	Calories	Cholesterol (mg)

FATS AND OILS

Product	Measure/ Quantity	Calories	Cholesterol (mg)
Bacon fat	1 tbsp	126	na
Beef tallow	1 tbsp	116	14
Butter	1 tbsp	123	36
Butter Blend (Blue Bonnet)	1 tbsp	90	5
Butter Blend (Country Morning)	1 tbsp	100	10
Chicken fat	1 tbsp	115	11
Goose fat	1 tbsp	115	13
Lard	1 tbsp	116	12
Margarine	1 tbsp	100	0
Margarine, stick (Blue Bonnet)	1 tbsp	100	0
Margarine, stick (Fleishmann's)	1 tbsp	100	0
Margarine, stick (Land O Lakes)	1 tbsp	100	0
Margarine, stick (Mazola)	1 tbsp	100	0
Margarine, squeeze (Fleishmann's)	1 tbsp	100	0
Margarine, diet (Blue Bonnet)	1 tbsp	50	0
Margarine, diet (Mazola)	1 tbsp	50	0
Margarine, whipped (Blue Bonnet)	1 tbsp	70	0
Shortening (Crisco)	1 tbsp	106	0
Shortening, Butter Flavored (Crisco)	1 tbsp	110	0
Spread (Blue Bonnet)	1 tbsp	80	0
Spread, corn oil, stick (Fleishmann's)	1 tbsp	80	0
Spread, whipped (Blue Bonnet)	1 tbsp	50	0
Turkey fat	1 tbsp	115	13
Vegetable oils (all)	1 tbsp	120	0

Product	Measure/ Quantity	Calories	Cholesterol (mg)
FISH			
Bass, striped, raw	3½ oz	105	80
Bluefish, broiled	3½ oz	147	73
Caviar, sturgeon	1 tsp	26	25
Chub, raw	3½ oz	145	50
Clams, raw	6 large	65	49
Clam juice	½ cup	19	13
Cod, broiled	3½ oz	162	na
Cod, dried, salted	3½ oz	130	82
Cod, raw	3½ oz	78	43
Crab, canned	½ cup	86	86
Crab, steamed	3½ oz	93	100
Eel, American, smoked	1¾ oz	165	35
Fish loaf	3½ oz	124	99
Fish sticks	4½ sticks	176	70
Flatfish, raw	3½ oz	79	61
Flounder, baked	3½ oz	202	na
Frog legs, raw	3½ oz	73	50
Haddock, fried	3½ oz	165	na
Haddock, raw	3½ oz	79	60
Halibut, raw	3½ oz	100	50
Halibut, broiled	3½ oz	171	60
Herring, raw	3½ oz	176	85
Herring, canned	3½ oz	208	98
Lobster, Atlantic, raw	3½ oz	191	95
Lobster, Northern, raw	3½ oz	91	95
Lobster, cooked	3½ oz	92	84
Mackerel, raw	3½ oz	191	95
Mackerel, broiled	3½ oz	231	100
Mackerel, canned	½ cup	192	107
Oysters, Eastern, raw	5-8 medium	66	49
Perch, raw	3½ oz	94	90
SALMON			
Atlantic, raw	3½ oz	217	35
Atlantic, canned	3½ oz	203	35
Chinook, canned	3½ oz	210	60

Product	Measure/ Quantity	Calories	Cholesterol (mg)
FISH			
Sockeye (red), raw	3½ oz	171	36
Sockeye (red), canned	3½ oz	171	36
Sockeye (red), broiled or baked	3½ oz	182	47
Sockeye (red), smoked	3½ oz	176	60
Sardines in oil	8	311	120
Scallops, raw	3½ oz	81	35
Scallops, steamed	3½ oz	112	53
Shrimp, raw	3½ oz	91	150
Shrimp, canned, wet pack	3½ oz	80	150
Shrimp, French fried	3½ oz	225	120
Sole	3½ oz	68	48
Sucker, carp, raw	3½ oz	na	0
Trout, brook, raw	3½ oz	101	55
Trout, rainbow, raw	3½ oz	195	55
TUNA			
Chunk Light in Oil (Chicken of the Sea)	½ cup	225	16
Chunk Light in Water (Chicken of the Sea)	½ cup	100	37
Chunk White in Oil (Chicken of the Sea)	½ cup	250	14
Chunk White in Water Low Sodium (Chicken of the Sea)	½ cup	110	22
Solid Light in Oil (Chicken of the Sea)	½ cup	230	16
Solid White in Oil (Chicken of the Sea)	½ cup	225	13
Solid White in Water (Chicken of the Sea)	½ cup	220	13

FLOUR AND GRAINS

Barley flour	1 cup	112	0
Barley, pearled, cooked	3½ oz	118	0
Barley, pearled, dry	3½ oz	343	0

Product	Measure/ Quantity	Calories	Cholesterol (mg)
FLOUR AND GRAINS			
Buckwheat groats, cooked	3½ oz	364	0
Buckwheat groats, dry	3½ oz	343	0
Corn bran	3½ oz	na	0
Corn meal, degermed	1 cup	454	0
Corn meal, whole grain	1 cup	433	0
Grits, cooked	1 cup	146	0
Millet, cooked	3½ oz	na	0
Millet, dry	3½ oz	327	0
Oat bran	¼ cup	58	0
Oat flour, milled	3½ oz	390	0
Oat flour, whole grain	3½ oz	347	0
Oats, rolled	1 cup	144	0
Popcorn, popped	4 cups	90	0
Rice, brown, cooked	1 cup	214	0
Rice, brown, dry	1 cup	707	0
Rice, Beef Flavored (Minute Rice)	½ cup	152	10
Rice, Chicken Flavored (Minute Rice)	½ cup	153	10
Rice, Chinese Style (Birds Eye)	½ cup	106	Tr
Rice, French Style (Birds Eye)	½ cup	118	0
Rice, Northern Italian Style (Birds Eye)	½ cup	111	3
Rice, Pilaf (Pritikin)	½ cup	90	0
Rice, Spanish (Minute Rice)	½ cup	150	10
Rice, Spanish (Pritikin)	½ cup	100	0
Rice, white, cooked	1 cup	200	0
Rice, white, dry	1 cup	712	0
Rice, wild, cooked	3½ oz	148	0
Rice flour	1 cup	479	0
Rye flour, light	1 cup	357	0
Rye flour, dark	1 cup	404	0
Soybean flour, defatted	1 cup	326	0
Wheat bran	3½ oz	198	0

Product	Measure/ Quantity	Calories	Cholesterol (mg)

FLOUR AND GRAINS

Product	Measure/Quantity	Calories	Cholesterol (mg)
Wheat germ	3½ oz	351	0
White, all-purpose	1 cup	400	0
White cake flour	1 cup	364	0
Whole wheat	1 cup	400	0

FRUIT

Note: All canned fruits are in heavy syrup unless otherwise indicated. All fresh fruits are unpeeled and raw unless otherwise indicated.

Product	Measure/Quantity	Calories	Cholesterol (mg)
Apple	1 lg	57	0
Apple, canned, unsweetened	½ cup	69	0
Applesauce, unsweetened	½ cup	53	0
Apricot	2	32	0
Avocado	½ med	153	0
Banana	1 med	96	0
Blackberries	½ cup	27	0
Blueberries, canned	½ cup	112	0
Blueberries, frozen	½ cup	93	0
Boysenberries, canned	½ cup	113	0
Boysenberries, frozen	½ cup	33	0
Cantaloupe	1 cup	39	0
Cherries	10	38	0
Cherries, canned, unsweetened	½ cup	64	0
Cranberries	½ cup	31	0
Cranberry sauce	2 oz	89	0
Currants, red, raw	½ cup	31	0
Dates, dried	4	98	0
Figs, dried	2	93	0
Fruit Cocktail (Libby's)	½ cup	85	0
Gooseberries	½ cup	34	0
Grapefruit	½ med	39	0
Grapefruit, canned, unsweetened	½ cup	46	0

Product	Measure/ Quantity	Calories	Cholesterol (mg)
	FRUIT		
Grapes, black	10	30	0
Grapes, white	10	36	0
Honeydew	1 cup	42	0
Mango	1 med	135	0
Nectarine	1 sm	44	0
Orange	1 med	65	0
Peach	1 med	37	0
Peaches, cling, canned, unsweetened	½ cup	54	0
Pear	1 med	98	0
Pears, canned	½ cup	94	0
Pineapple	½ cup	39	0
Pineapple, canned (Dole)	½ cup	95	0
Plums	3 sm	38	0
Prunes	2	37	0
Raisins	½ cup	225	0
Raspberries	½ cup	42	0
Rhubarb, cooked	3½ oz	9	0
Strawberry	1 lg	35	0
Strawberries, canned, unsweetened	½ cup	26	0
Tangerine	1 lg	39	0
Watermelon	1 cup	35	0
	GOOSE		
Flesh and skin, raw	3½ oz	371	80
Flesh only, roasted	3½ oz	238	96
Flesh and skin, roasted	3½ oz	305	91
Liver pâté	2 oz	262	86
	HOT DOGS		
Chicken frankfurter	1	116	45
Chicken Franks (Tyson)	3½ oz	285	68
Chicken Corn Dogs (Tyson)	3½ oz	280	55
Corn Dogs (Oscar Mayer)	1	330	37

Product	Measure/ Quantity	Calories	Cholesterol (mg)
HOT DOGS			
Frankfurter, beef	1	142	27
Franks, Beef (Oscar Mayer)	1	145	27
Hot Dog (Armour)	1	150	20
Turkey frankfurters	1	102	48
Turkey Franks (Louis Rich)	1	100	39
Weiners (Oscar Mayer)	1	145	24
Weiners with Cheese (Oscar Mayer)	1	145	31

ICE CREAM AND FROZEN DESSERTS

Product	Measure/ Quantity	Calories	Cholesterol (mg)
Frozfruit, pineapple	1	68	0
Pudding Pops, banana	1	90	1
Ice cream, vanilla, 10% fat	½ cup	135	30
Ice cream, vanilla, 16% fat	½ cup	175	44
Ice Cream, Vanilla (Land O Lakes)	½ cup	140	30
Ice Milk, Vanilla (Land O Lakes)	½ cup	90	10
Sherbet, orange	½ cup	135	7

JAM, SUGAR, AND SYRUP

Product	Measure/ Quantity	Calories	Cholesterol (mg)
Honey	1 tbsp	61	0
Jam, plum	1 tbsp	55	0
Jam, strawberry	1 tbsp	55	0
Maple syrup	1 tbsp	50	0
Maple Syrup, Buttered (Log Cabin)	1 tbsp	60	1
Marmalade	1 tbsp	56	0
Sugar, white	1 tbsp	46	0
Sweet 'n Low	1 pkg	4	0

Product	Measure/ Quantity	Calories	Cholesterol (mg)

LAMB

Note: All figures are for separable lean only.

Product	Measure/ Quantity	Calories	Cholesterol (mg)
All cuts, raw	3½ oz	262	70
Arm chop, lean, broiled	3½ oz	339	81
Blade chop, lean, roasted	3½ oz	340	81
Leg, lean, roasted	3½ oz	242	99
Rib chop, lean, cooked	3½ oz	423	98

MILK AND MILK BEVERAGES

Product	Measure/ Quantity	Calories	Cholesterol (mg)
CREAM			
Half and half	½ cup	158	45
Light	½ cup	235	80
Medium	½ cup	292	105
Nondairy Creamer (Coffee-Mate)	1 tsp	11	<1
Nondairy Creamer (Coffee-Rich)	½ oz	22	0
Nondairy Creamer (Cremora)	1 tsp	12	0
Sour	½ cup	247	51
Sour, nondairy imitation	½ cup	240	0
Whipping (heavy)	½ cup	411	163
Whipped Topping (nondairy)	½ cup	120	0
Whipped Topping Mix (D-Zerta)	½ cup	64	3
MILK			
Buttermilk, cultured	1 cup	99	9
Buttermilk, dry	1 tbsp	25	5
Condensed sweetened	½ cup	492	52
Evaporated, skim	½ cup	100	4
Evaporated, whole (Carnation)	½ cup	170	37
Goat milk	1 cup	168	28
Human milk	1 cup	168	32

Product	Measure/ Quantity	Calories	Cholesterol (mg)

MILK AND MILK BEVERAGES

Product	Measure/Quantity	Calories	Cholesterol (mg)
Lowfat, 1% fat	1 cup	102	10
Lowfat, 2% fat	1 cup	121	18
Skim	1 cup	86	4
Skim, Dry, Instant (Carnation)	1 cup prepared	80	4
Soybean milk	1 cup	87	0
Soybean Milk, Soyamel	1 cup	130	0
Whole, 3.3% fat	1 cup	150	33
Whole, 3.5% fat	1 cup	150	34
Whole, 3.7% fat	1 cup	157	35

MILK BEVERAGES

Note: Unless otherwise noted, all milk drinks are listed as prepared with 1 cup whole milk.

Product	Measure/Quantity	Calories	Cholesterol (mg)
Chocolate (Nestlé Quik)	1 cup	240	33
Chocolate (Ovaltine)	1 cup	230	33
Egg nog, nonalcoholic	1 cup	342	149
Hot Cocoa, prep. w/water (Carnation)	1 cup	110	2
Hot Cocoa, prep. w/water (Swiss Miss)	1 cup	147	0
Hot Cocoa, 70 Calorie, prepared w/water (Carnation)	1 cup	70	2
Instant Breakfast, Vanilla (Carnation)	1 cup	280	38
Malted milk	1 cup	236	37
Chocolate Malted milk (Carnation)	1 cup	235	35
Milkshake, homemade	1 cup	421	na

NUTS AND PEANUT BUTTER

Product	Measure/Quantity	Calories	Cholesterol (mg)
Almonds	24–30	180	0
Beechnuts	1 oz	171	0
Brazils	8 med	194	0

Product	Measure/ Quantity	Calories	Cholesterol (mg)
NUTS AND PEANUT BUTTER			
Cashews	6–8 nuts	84	0
Chestnuts	6 sm	58	0
Coconut, shredded, sweetened	2 tbsp	53	0
Hazelnuts (filberts)	10–12	97	0
Hickory nuts	15 small	101	0
Litchi	6	45	0
Macadamia nuts	6	109	0
Peanuts	1 oz	152	0
Peanut Butter, smooth (Jif)	2 tbsp	186	0
Pecans	12	208	0
Pignolias	2 tbsp	84	0
Pistachios	30	88	0
Walnuts, black	4–5	98	0
PANCAKES AND WAFFLES			
French Toast (Downyflake)	2 slices	270	<5
Pancakes, from batter (Mrs. Smith's)	3, 4″ each	230	40
Pancakes (Downyflake)	2 oz	160	<5
Pancakes, Blueberry (Aunt Jemima)	3	260	<5
Pancakes, Microwave (Pillsbury)	3	240	<5
Pancakes, from mix	4″	159	54
Waffles, from mix	1	205	45
Waffles, toaster (Eggo)	2	240	0
Waffles, toaster, whole wheat (Eggo)	2	260	0
Waffles, toaster, whole wheat (Roman Meal)	2	280	<5

Product	Measure/ Quantity	Calories	Cholesterol (mg)

PASTA

Note: All items in this category are cooked.

Product	Measure/ Quantity	Calories	Cholesterol (mg)
Egg noodles	1 cup	200	50
Macaroni and Spaghetti (Ronzoni)	1 cup	210	0
Spinach Linguini (Buitoni)	1 cup	210	0
Superoni (Prince)	1 cup	210	0
Whole wheat (100%)	1 cup	207	0

PASTRY

Product	Measure/ Quantity	Calories	Cholesterol (mg)
Crepes, Apple (Mrs. Smith's)	1	195	15
Crepes, Strawberry (Mrs. Smith's)	1	150	15
Cream Puffs, Chocolate, frozen (Rich's)	1	145	23
Cream puffs, homemade	1	245	187
Danish, Apple (Hostess)	1	360	19
Danish, Butterhorn (Hostess)	1	330	8
Danish, Raspberry (Hostess)	1	300	20
Donuts, Bavarian Creme (Morton)	1	180	11
Donuts, Cinnamon (Hostess)	1	110	6
Donuts, Chocolate Iced (Morton)	1	150	10
Donuts, Jelly (Morton)	1	180	11
Donuts, Old Fashioned (Hostess)	1	180	9
Donuts, Old Fashioned Glazed (Hostess)	1	230	11
Donuts, Powdered Sugar (Hostess)	1	110	6

Product	Measure/ Quantity	Calories	Cholesterol (mg)
PASTRY			
Eclair, Chocolate, frozen			
(Rich's)	1	234	60
Honey Buns (Hostess)	1	450	24
Popovers, homemade	1	112	59
Pop Tarts, Blueberry	1	210	0
Pop Tarts, Strawberry			
Frosted	1	200	0
Streusel, Apple	½ pack-		
(Mrs. Smith's)	age	420	5
Toastettes, Apple	1	190	0
Toastettes, Brown Sugar			
Cinnamon	1	190	0
PIES			
DESSERT PIES			
Apple (Morton)	4 oz slice	289	12
Apple (Mrs. Smith's)	⅛ pie	390	10
Apple, Old Fashioned			
(Mrs. Smith's)	⅛ pie	515	10
Banana Cream			
(Mrs. Smith's)	⅛ pie	240	5
Blueberry (Morton)	4 oz slice	280	12
Blueberry (Mrs. Smith's)	⅛ pie	380	10
Cherry (Morton)	4 oz slice	300	12
Cherry (Mrs. Smith's)	⅛ pie	400	10
Cherry Lattice			
(Mrs. Smith's)	⅛ pie	350	5
Cherry Natural Juice			
(Mrs. Smith's)	⅛ pie	350	5
Chocolate Cream			
(Mrs. Smith's)	⅛ pie	270	5
Coconut Cream			
(Mrs. Smith's)	⅛ pie	270	5

Product	Measure/ Quantity	Calories	Cholesterol (mg)
PIES			
Coconut Custard	⅛ pie	330	50
Custard, homemade	⅙ pie	327	160
Custard (Mrs. Smith's)	⅛ pie	300	65
Lemon chiffon pie, homemade, made with lard	⅙ pie	335	183
Lemon Cream (Mrs. Smith's)	⅛ pie	245	5
Lemon meringue pie, homemade, made with lard	⅙ pie	350	130
Lemon Meringue (Mrs. Smith's)	⅛ pie	310	35
Mince (Morton)	4 oz slice	310	12
Peach (Morton)	4 oz slice	280	12
Peach (Mrs. Smith's)	⅛ pie	365	10
Pecan (Mrs. Smith's)	⅛ pie	510	30
Pumpkin (Morton)	4 oz slice	230	44
Pumpkin Custard (Mrs. Smith's)	⅛ pie	310	30
SNACK PIES			
Apple (Hostess)	1 pie	390	18
Blueberry (Hostess)	1 pie	390	18
Cherry (Hostess)	1 pie	390	18
Lemon (Hostess)	1 pie	400	30

PORK

Note: Fresh meat figures are for separable lean only, unless otherwise mentioned.

BACON	2 slices	73	11
Farmland	2 slices	84	9
Oscar Mayer	2 slices	70	10

Product	Measure/ Quantity	Calories	Cholesterol (mg)
PORK			
Bacon Bits (Oscar Mayer)	½ oz	40	12
Brains, cooked	3½ oz	138	2551
Breakfast Strips (Oscar Mayer)	2 strips	90	20
Brown 'n Serve Links (Swift)	2 links	190	35
Brown 'n Serve Patties (Swift)	2 patties	190	40
Canadian Bacon (Oscar Mayer)	2 oz	80	24
Chitterlings, raw	3½ oz	249	158
Chitterlings, cooked	3½ oz	304	144
Ears, cooked	1 ear	183	99
Feet, cooked	3½ oz	193	99
HAM			
Boneless, smoked (Oscar Mayer)	3½ oz	175	58
Fresh, raw	3½ oz	137	57
Fresh, roasted	3½ oz	312	133
Canned (Oscar Mayer)	3½ oz	110	41
Canned (Swift Premium)	3½ oz	190	70
Ham steaks (Oscar Mayer)	3½ oz	120	46
Ham patties	2 patties	406	86
Heart, braised	3½ oz	148	221
Kidneys, braised	3½ oz	151	480
Loin, raw	3½ oz	156	60
Loin, broiled	3½ oz	256	95
Loin, roasted	3½ oz	240	91
Shoulder, raw	3½ oz	154	67
Shoulder, roasted	3½ oz	244	96
Sirloin, broiled	3½ oz	244	98
Sirloin, raw	3½ oz	151	63
Spareribs, braised, lean and fat	3½ oz	398	121
Spareribs, raw, lean and fat	3½ oz	284	77
Tenderloin, raw	3½ oz	112	63

Product	Measure/ Quantity	Calories	Cholesterol (mg)
PORK			
Tenderloin, roasted	3½ oz	166	93
Tongue, braised	3½ oz	271	146
Top loin, broiled	3½ oz	258	94
Top loin, fried	3½ oz	258	81
Top loin, raw	3½ oz	161	55
Sizzlean (Swift)	2 strips	70	20
POTATO CHIPS AND SNACKS			
Cheez Curls (Planters)	1 oz	160	5
Corn Chips (Planters)	1 oz	160	0
Fritos	1 oz	150	0
Popcorn	4 cups	90	0
Potato Chips (Wise)	1 oz	160	0
Potato Crunchies (Planters)	1 oz	152	0
Pretzels (Mr. Salty)	1 oz	110	0
Pretzels (Rold Gold)	1 oz	110	0
Tortilla chips (Buenos)	1 oz	150	0
PUDDING			
Banana Pudding (Jell-O)	½ cup	160	18
Banana Pudding, Instant (Jell-O)	½ cup	170	16
Banana Pudding (Royal)	½ cup	160	14
Banana Pudding, Instant (Royal)	½ cup	180	15
Blancmange, homemade	½ cup	143	18
Butterscotch Pudding (Jell-O)	½ cup	170	16
Butterscotch Pudding, Instant (Jell-O)	½ cup	170	16
Butterscotch Pudding (Royal)	½ cup	160	15
Butterscotch Pudding, Instant (Royal)	½ cup	180	15

Product	Measure/ Quantity	Calories	Cholesterol (mg)

PUDDING

Product	Measure/ Quantity	Calories	Cholesterol (mg)
Chocolate pudding, homemade	½ cup	193	15
Chocolate Pudding (Jell-O)	½ cup	160	16
Chocolate Pudding, Instant (Jell-O)	½ cup	180	16
Chocolate Pudding (My-T-Fine)	½ cup	133	169
Chocolate Pudding (Royal)	½ cup	180	15
Chocolate Pudding, Instant (Royal)	½ cup	190	15
Chocolate Pudding, Reduced Calorie (D-Zerta)	½ cup	60	2
Chocolate Fudge Pudding (Jell-O)	½ cup	160	17
Chocolate Fudge Pudding, Instant (Jell-O)	½ cup	180	17
Coconut Pudding, Instant (Royal)	½ cup	170	15
Corn pudding, homemade	½ cup	119	52
Custard, homemade	½ cup	153	139
Custard (Jell-O Americana)	½ cup	160	81
Custard (Royal)	½ cup	150	15
Flan (Royal)	½ cup	150	15
Key Lime Pie Filling (Royal)	½ cup	160	135
Lemon Pudding (Jell-O)	½ cup	170	93
Lemon Pudding, Instant	½ cup	178	13
Lemon Pudding, Instant (Royal)	½ cup	180	15
Milk Chocolate Pudding (Jell-O)	½ cup	170	17
Milk Chocolate Pudding, Instant (Jell-O)	½ cup	180	17
Pineapple Cream Pudding, Instant (Jell-O)	½ cup	170	16
Pistachio Pudding, Instant (Jell-O)	½ cup	180	17

Product	Measure/ Quantity	Calories	Cholesterol (mg)
PUDDING			
Rice pudding	½ cup	175	15
Tapioca, from mix	½ cup	170	17
Tapioca (Jell-O)	½ cup	160	16
Vanilla Pudding (Jell-O)	½ cup	160	16
Vanilla Pudding (Royal)	½ cup	160	15
Vanilla Pudding, Reduced Calorie (D-Zerta)	½ cup	70	2

SALAD DRESSING

Product	Measure/ Quantity	Calories	Cholesterol (mg)
REDUCED CALORIE			
Blue Cheese (Roka)	1 tbsp	14	5
Blue Cheese, Chunky (Kraft)	1 tbsp	30	0
Buttermilk (Kraft)	1 tbsp	30	0
Cucumber, Creamy (Kraft)	1 tbsp	30	0
French	1 tbsp	22	1
French (Kraft)	1 tbsp	20	0
French Style (Pritikin)	1 tbsp	10	0
Italian	1 tbsp	16	1
Italian (Kraft)	1 tbsp	6	0
Italian (Pritikin)	1 tbsp	6	0
Italian, Creamy (Kraft)	1 tbsp	25	0
Italian, Oil-Free (Kraft)	1 tbsp	4	0
Russian	1 tbsp	23	1
Russian (Kraft)	1 tbsp	30	0
Russian (Pritikin)	1 tbsp	18	0
Thousand Island	1 tbsp	24	2
Thousand Island (Kraft)	1 tbsp	30	5
Vinaigrette (Pritikin)	1 tbsp	10	0
Zesty Tomato (Pritikin)	1 tbsp	18	0
REGULAR			
Bacon & Buttermilk (Kraft)	1 tbsp	80	0
Blue Cheese (Roka)	1 tbsp	60	10

Product	Measure/ Quantity	Calories	Cholesterol (mg)

SALAD DRESSING

Product	Measure/ Quantity	Calories	Cholesterol (mg)
Blue Cheese, Chunky (Kraft)	1 tbsp	70	0
Blue Cheese, Chunky (Wish-Bone)	1 tbsp	70	0
Blue Cheese, from mix	1 tbsp	84	Tr
Blue Cheese, from mix (Good Seasons)	1 tbsp	84	5
Buttermilk, Creamy (Kraft)	1 tbsp	80	5
Buttermilk, from mix (Good Seasons)	1 tbsp	58	5
Buttermilk & Chives, Creamy (Kraft)	1 tbsp	80	5
Caesar (Wish-Bone)	1 tbsp	80	0
Coleslaw (Kraft)	1 tbsp	70	15
Cucumber, Creamy (Kraft)	1 tbsp	70	0
Cucumber (Philadelphia)	1 tbsp	70	0
Farm Style, from mix (Good Seasons)	1 tbsp	53	4
French, from mix	1 tbsp	97	8
French, Catalina	1 tbsp	60	0
French, Garlic (Wish-Bone)	1 tbsp	60	0
French, Kraft	1 tbsp	60	0
French, Old Fashioned, from mix (Good Seasons)	1 tbsp	84	0
French, Riviera, from mix (Good Seasons)	1 tbsp	91	0
French, Sweet & Spicy (Wish-Bone)	1 tbsp	60	0
Garlic, from mix	1 tbsp	83	0
Garlic (Wish-Bone)	1 tbsp	80	0
Garlic & Chive (Philadelphia)	1 tbsp	70	0

Product	Measure/ Quantity	Calories	Cholesterol (mg)

SALAD DRESSING

Product	Measure/ Quantity	Calories	Cholesterol (mg)
Garlic with cheese, from mix	1 tbsp	85	Tr
Italian, from mix	1 tbsp	84	0
Italian Herb (Philadelphia)	1 tbsp	70	0
Italian, Golden Blend (Kraft)	1 tbsp	70	0
Italian, mild, from mix	1 tbsp	84	0
Italian with cheese, from mix	1 tbsp	88	Tr
Italian, Zesty (Kraft)	1 tbsp	80	0
Oil and Vinegar, homemade	1 tbsp	72	0
Oil & Vinegar (Kraft)	1 tbsp	70	0
Onion, from mix	1 tbsp	85	0
Onion & Chives, creamy (Kraft)	1 tbsp	70	0
Russian (Kraft)	1 tbsp	60	0
Sesame seed	1 tbsp	68	0
Spin blend	1 tbsp	50	8
Thousand Island (Kraft)	1 tbsp	70	10
Toasted Onion (Philadelphia)	1 tbsp	70	0

SANDWICH MEATS

Product	Measure/ Quantity	Calories	Cholesterol (mg)
Barbecue Loaf (Armour)	2 oz	100	20
Bar-B-Q Loaf (Oscar Mayer)	2 oz	90	22
Beef, Smoked (Buddig)	2 oz	78	32
Beef, Spicy (Land O' Frost)	2 oz	80	24
BOLOGNA			
Beef	2 oz	176	33
Beef (Armour)	2 oz	180	30
Beef (Oscar Mayer)	2 oz	184	32
Beef & Pork (Armour)	2 oz	180	30

Product	Measure/ Quantity	Calories	Cholesterol (mg)

SANDWICH MEATS

Product	Measure/ Quantity	Calories	Cholesterol (mg)
Beef & Pork (Oscar Mayer)	2 oz	184	32
Berliner	2 oz	130	26
Bologna & Cheese (Oscar Mayer)	2 oz	184	34
Chicken Bologna (Tyson)	2 oz	130	34
Lebanon Bologna	2 oz	128	38
Turkey Bologna	2 oz	113	56
Turkey Bologna (Armour)	2 oz	110	95
Braunschweiger (Oscar Mayer)	2 oz	190	78
Chicken Roll, Breast (Tyson)	2 oz	88	27
Chicken roll, light meat	2 oz	90	28
Chicken, Smoked (Buddig)	2 oz	94	24
Chicken spread	2 oz	110	na
Corn Beef, Cooked (Buddig)	2 oz	78	32
Corned beef	2 oz	142	55
Corned Beef (Land O' Frost)	2 oz	80	24
Corned beef, canned	2 oz	141	49
Corned beef loaf	2 oz	86	26
Corned Beef Loaf (Oscar Mayer)	2 oz	90	26
Dried beef	2 oz	94	na
Dutch Brand Loaf	2 oz	136	26
Ham, Chopped (Oscar Mayer)	2 oz	130	28
Ham, Cooked (Oscar Mayer)	2 oz	67	27
Ham, Smoked (Buddig)	2 oz	96	40
Ham & Cheese Loaf (Oscar Mayer)	2 oz	150	32
Ham and cheese spread	2 oz	138	34
Ham salad spread	2 oz	122	20
Head Cheese (Oscar Mayer)	2 oz	110	50

| | Measure/ | | Cholesterol |
| Product | Quantity | Calories | (mg) |

SANDWICH MEATS

Product	Measure/Quantity	Calories	Cholesterol (mg)
Honey Loaf (Oscar Mayer)	2 oz	70	20
Liver Cheese (Oscar Mayer)	2 oz	171	103
Liverwurst (Armour)	2 oz	180	90
Liverwurst spread	½ can	220	na
Luncheon meat, beef	2 oz	70	24
Luncheon meat, pork and beef	2 oz	200	30
Luncheon meat, pork, canned	2 oz	190	36
Luncheon Roll Sausage (Oscar Mayer)	2 oz	86	29
Luxury Loaf (Oscar Mayer)	2 oz	80	22
Mother's Loaf	2 oz	160	26
Old Fashioned Loaf (Armour)	2 oz	160	30
Old Fashioned Loaf (Oscar Mayer)	2 oz	130	26
Olive Loaf (Armour)	2 oz	140	20
Pastrami	2 oz	198	52
Pastrami, Smoked (Buddig)	2 oz	78	32
Peppered Loaf (Oscar Mayer)	2 oz	80	28
Pickle & Pimiento Loaf (Armour)	2 oz	160	20
Pickle & Pimiento Loaf (Oscar Mayer)	2 oz	130	22
Picnic loaf	2 oz	132	22
Poultry salad spread	2 oz	114	18
Pressed Luncheon Sausage (Oscar Mayer)	2 oz	86	34
SALAMI			
Beef	2 oz	148	36
Beef, beer salami	2 oz	186	34
Cooked (Armour)	2 oz	160	40
Cotto (Oscar Mayer)	2 oz	123	34
Cotto, Beef (Oscar Mayer)	2 oz	123	34

Product	Measure/ Quantity	Calories	Cholesterol (mg)
SANDWICH MEATS			
Genoa (Armour)	2 oz	220	60
Hard (Armour)	2 oz	240	40
Hard (Oscar Mayer)	2 oz	220	44
Salami for Beer (Oscar Mayer)	2 oz	135	32
Turkey Cotto Salami (Armour)	2 oz	90	35
Turkey Cotto Salami (Louis Rich)	2 oz	100	46
Turkey salami	2 oz	112	47
Sandwich Spread (Oscar Mayer)	2 oz	130	20
Spiced Luncheon Meat (Armour)	2 oz	180	40
Turkey (Land O' Frost)	2 oz	100	23
Turkey Breast (Longacre)	2 oz	60	20
Turkey Breast, Smoked (Louis Rich)	2 oz	54	16
Turkey Ham (Armour)	2 oz	70	30
Turkey Ham (Land O' Frost)	2 oz	70	23
Turkey Ham (Louis Rich)	2 oz	80	34
Turkey loaf, breast meat	2 oz	62	23
Turkey Pastrami (Armour)	2 oz	70	33
Turkey Pastrami (Louis Rich)	2 oz	70	30
Turkey roll, light meat	2 oz	84	24
Turkey roll, light and dark	2 oz	84	32
Turkey Roll, white (Magic Slice)	2 oz	80	17
Turkey Roll, white & dark (Magic Slice)	2 oz	80	17
Turkey, Smoked (Buddig)	2 oz	90	12
Turkey, Smoked (Louis Rich)	2 oz	60	24

Product	Measure/ Quantity	Calories	Cholesterol (mg)
SAUSAGE			
Beef, smoked	1 link	134	29
Beef Smokies (Oscar Mayer)	1 link	130	30
Blood sausage	2 oz	214	68
Bratwurst	1 link	256	51
Breakfast Links, Vegetarian (Morningstar Farms)	3 links	180	0
Breakfast Sausage (Jimmy Dean)	2 oz	227	48
Brotwurst	1 link	226	44
Cheese Smokies (Oscar Mayer)	1 link	140	30
Country style	3 links	144	33
German Sausage (Armour)	2 oz	180	40
Ham Roll Sausage (Oscar Mayer)	2 oz	86	27
Honey roll sausage	2 oz	104	28
Hot Mett (Hillshire Farms)	2 oz	181	31
Italian sausage	1 link	217	52
Kielbasa	2 oz	184	40
Kielbasa (Hillshire Farms)	2 oz	183	32
Knockwurst	1 link	209	39
Little Friers (Oscar Mayer)	2 links	160	36
Mortadella	2 oz	176	32
New England Brand (Oscar Mayer)	2 oz	70	28
Pepperoni (Armour)	2 oz	260	40
Sausage Patties (Oscar Mayer)	1 patty	125	27
Smoked Sausage (Kahn's)	2 oz	181	31
Smokie Links (Oscar Mayer)	1 link	135	26
Summer sausage	2 oz	190	42
Summer Sausage (Oscar Mayer)	2 oz	184	42
Summer Sausage, Beef (Oscar Mayer)	2 oz	172	42

Product	Measure/ Quantity	Calories	Cholesterol (mg)
SAUSAGE			
Turkey Breakfast Sausage (Louis Rich)	2 oz	130	46
Turkey Smoked Sausage (Louis Rich)	2 oz	110	38
Turkey Summer Sausage (Louis Rich)	2 oz	100	44
Vienna Sausage	6	270	48
SOUP			
CANNED SOUPS			
Bean with bacon	8 fl oz	173	3
Bean with Bacon (Campbell's)	8 fl oz	150	5
Bean with frankfurters	8 fl oz	187	12
Bean with ham, chunky	8 fl oz	231	22
Beef (Campbell's)	8 fl oz	80	10
Beef broth	8 fl oz	16	Tr
Beef Broth (Campbell's)	8 fl oz	16	0
Beef, chunky	8 fl oz	171	14
Beef and mushroom	8 fl oz	72	7
Beef noodle	8 fl oz	84	5
Beef Noodle (Campbell's)	8 fl oz	70	11
Beef Noodle, Homestyle (Campbell's)	8 fl oz	80	16
Beef vegetable with barley	8 fl oz	79	5
Beefy Mushroom (Campbell's)	8 fl oz	60	7
Black bean	8 fl oz	116	0
Black Bean (Campbell's)	8 fl oz	110	0
Cheddar Cheese (Campbell's)	8 fl oz	130	11
Cheese	8 fl oz	155	30
Cheese, prepared with milk	8 fl oz	230	48

Product	Measure/ Quantity	Calories	Cholesterol (mg)
SOUP			
Chicken Alphabet (Campbell's)	8 fl oz	70	6
Chicken and dumplings	8 fl oz	97	34
Chicken broth	8 fl oz	39	1
Chicken Broth (Campbell's)	8 fl oz	35	0
Chicken Broth (Pritikin)	6⅞ fl oz	14	0
Chicken Broth and Noodles (Campbell's)	8 fl oz	60	9
Chicken Broth with Rice (Campbell's)	8 fl oz	50	0
Chicken, chunky	8 fl oz	178	30
Chicken 'N Dumplings (Campbell's)	8 fl oz	80	22
Chicken gumbo	8 fl oz	56	5
Chicken Gumbo (Campbell's)	8 fl oz	60	4
Chicken mushroom	8 fl oz	na	10
Chicken noodle	8 fl oz	75	7
Chicken Noodle (Campbell's)	8 fl oz	70	14
Chicken noodle, chunky	8 fl oz	180	18
Chicken Noodle, Homestyle (Campbell's)	8 fl oz	70	14
Chicken noodle with meatballs	8 fl oz	99	10
Chicken NoodleOs (Campbell's)	8 fl oz	70	19
Chicken with Ribbon Pasta (Pritikin)	7¼ fl oz	60	0
Chicken rice	8 fl oz	60	7
Chicken Rice (Campbell's)	8 fl oz	60	7
Chicken rice, chunky	8 fl oz	127	12
Chicken and Stars (Campbell's)	8 fl oz	60	8
Chicken vegetable	8 fl oz	74	10

Product	Measure/ Quantity	Calories	Cholesterol (mg)
	SOUP		
Chicken Vegetable (Campbell's)	8 fl oz	70	10
Chicken Vegetable (Pritikin)	7¼ fl oz	70	0
Chicken vegetable, chunky	8 fl oz	167	17
Chili beef	8 fl oz	169	12
Chili Beef (Campbell's)	8 fl oz	130	11
Clam chowder, Manhattan	8 fl oz	78	2
Clam Chowder, Manhattan (Campbell's)	8 fl oz	70	0
Clam chowder, Manhattan, chunky	8 fl oz	133	14
Clam chowder, New England	8 fl oz	95	5
Clam Chowder, New England (Campbell's)	8 fl oz	80	5
Clam Chowder, New England, prepared with milk	8 fl oz	163	22
Clam Chowder, New England	8 fl oz	150	22
Consommé, beef	8 fl oz	29	0
Consommé, Beef (Campbell's)	8 fl oz	25	0
Crab	8 fl oz	76	10
Cream of asparagus	8 fl oz	87	5
Cream of Asparagus (Campbell's)	8 fl oz	90	1
Cream of asparagus, prepared with milk	8 fl oz	161	22
Cream of Celery (Campbell's)	8 fl oz	90	15

Product	Measure/ Quantity	Calories	Cholesterol (mg)
SOUP			
Cream of celery, prepared with milk	8 fl oz	165	32
Cream of chicken	8 fl oz	116	10
Cream of Chicken (Campbell's)	8 fl oz	110	9
Cream of chicken, prepared with milk	8 fl oz	191	27
Creamy Chicken Mushroom (Campbell's)	8 fl oz	120	12
Cream of mushroom	8 fl oz	129	2
Cream of Mushroom (Campbell's)	8 fl oz	100	0
Cream of mushroom, prepared with milk	8 fl oz	203	20
Cream of onion	8 fl oz	100	15
Cream of Onion (Campbell's)	8 fl oz	100	15
Cream of onion, prepared with milk	8 fl oz	144	32
Cream of potato	8 fl oz	73	5
Cream of Potato (Campbell's)	8 fl oz	70	4
Cream of potato, prepared with milk	8 fl oz	148	22
Cream of shrimp	8 fl oz	90	17
Cream of Shrimp (Campbell's)	8 fl oz	90	20
Cream of shrimp, prepared with milk	8 fl oz	165	35
Cream of Shrimp, prepared with milk (Campbell's)	8 fl oz	160	37
Cream of Tomato, prepared with milk (Campbell's)	8 fl oz	110	18
Curly Noodle with Chicken (Campbell's)	8 fl oz	70	14

Product	Measure/ Quantity	Calories	Cholesterol (mg)
SOUP			
Escarole	8 fl oz	27	2
French Onion (Campbell's)	8 fl oz	60	1
Gazpacho	8 fl oz	57	0
Green Pea (Campbell's)	8 fl oz	160	3
Lentil with ham	8 fl oz	140	7
Meatball Alphabet (Campbell's)	8 fl oz	100	9
Minestrone	8 fl oz	83	2
Minestrone (Campbell's)	8 fl oz	80	0
Minestrone, chunky	8 fl oz	127	5
Mushroom barley	8 fl oz	50	0
Mushroom with beef stock	8 fl oz	85	7
Noodles & Ground Beef (Campbell's)	8 fl oz	90	22
Onion	8 fl oz	57	0
Oyster stew	8 fl oz	59	14
Oyster Stew (Campbell's)	8 fl oz	80	24
Oyster stew, prepared with milk	8 fl oz	134	32
Oyster Stew, prepared with milk (Campbell's)	8 fl oz	150	41
Pea, green	8 fl oz	164	0
Pea, green, prepared with milk	8 fl oz	239	18
Pepperpot	8 fl oz	103	10
Pepper Pot (Campbell's)	8 fl oz	90	37
Scotch broth	8 fl oz	80	5
Scotch Broth (Campbell's)	8 fl oz	160	4
Stockpot	8 fl oz	100	5
Tomato	8 fl oz	86	0
Tomato (Campbell's)	8 fl oz	90	0
Tomato (Pritikin)	7¼ fl oz	70	0
Tomato, prepared with milk	8 fl oz	160	17

Product	Measure/ Quantity	Calories	Cholesterol (mg)
		SOUP	
Tomato, prepared with milk (Campbell's)	8 fl oz	160	17
Tomato beef with noodle	8 fl oz	140	5
Tomato bisque	8 fl oz	123	4
Tomato Bisque (Campbell's)	8 fl oz	120	1
Tomato bisque, prepared with milk	8 fl oz	198	22
Tomato rice	8 fl oz	120	2
Tomato Rice, Old Fashioned (Campbell's)	8 fl oz	110	0
Turkey, chunky	8 fl oz	136	9
Turkey noodle	8 fl oz	69	5
Turkey Noodle (Campbell's)	8 fl oz	70	11
Turkey vegetable	8 fl oz	74	2
Turkey Vegetable (Campbell's)	8 fl oz	70	6
Vegetable (Campbell's)	8 fl oz	90	0
Vegetable (Pritikin)	7¼ fl oz	70	0
Vegetable beef	8 fl oz	79	5
Vegetable Beef (Campbell's)	8 fl oz	70	7
Vegetable with beef broth	8 fl oz	81	2
Vegetable, chunky	8 fl oz	122	0
Vegetable, Crispy Spanish Style (Campbell's)	8 fl oz	45	0
Vegetable, Homestyle (Campbell's)	8 fl oz	60	0
Vegetable, Old Fashioned (Campbell's)	8 fl oz	60	0
Vegetable, vegetarian	8 fl oz	72	0
Vegetable, Vegetarian (Campbell's)	8 fl oz	90	0
Vichyssoise	8 fl oz	148	22
Won Ton (Campbell's)	8 fl oz	40	10

Product	Measure/ Quantity	Calories	Cholesterol (mg)

SOUP

DRY SOUPS

Product	Measure/ Quantity	Calories	Cholesterol (mg)
Bean with bacon	8 fl oz	105	3
Beef bouillon	8 fl oz	19	1
Beef bouillon, cubed	8 fl oz	8	Tr
Beef noodle	8 fl oz	41	2
Cauliflower	8 fl oz	68	Tr
Chicken bouillon, cubed	8 fl oz	13	1
Chicken broth	8 fl oz	21	1
Chicken noodle	8 fl oz	53	3
Chicken rice	8 fl oz	60	3
Chicken vegetable	8 fl oz	49	3
Clam chowder, Manhattan	8 fl oz	65	Tr
Clam chowder, New England	8 fl oz	95	1
Consommé	8 fl oz	17	0
Cream of asparagus	8 fl oz	59	Tr
Cream of celery	8 fl oz	63	1
Cream of chicken	8 fl oz	107	3
Cream of vegetable	8 fl oz	105	0
Leek	8 fl oz	71	3
Minestrone	8 fl oz	79	3
Mushroom	8 fl oz	96	1
Onion	8 fl oz	28	0
Oxtail	8 fl oz	71	3
Split pea	8 fl oz	133	3
Tomato	8 fl oz	102	1
Tomato vegetable	8 fl oz	55	Tr
Vegetable beef	8 fl oz	53	1

TOMATOES AND TOMATO PRODUCTS

Product	Measure/ Quantity	Calories	Cholesterol (mg)
Canned, Whole (Hunt's)	½ cup	24	0
Fresh, cooked	½ cup	20	0
Marinara Sauce (Ragu)	½ cup	90	0
Mexican Sauce (Pritikin)	½ cup	50	0
Paste (Contadina)	¼ cup	50	0
Pizza Quick Sauce, Chunky	3 tbsp	45	0

Product	Measure/ Quantity	Calories	Cholesterol (mg)
TOMATOES AND TOMATO PRODUCTS			
Raw	1 small	18	0
Sauce (Del Monte)	½ cup	39	0
Spaghetti Sauce (Pritikin)	½ cup	60	0
Spaghetti Sauce with Mushrooms (Pritikin)	½ cup	60	0
Spaghetti Sauce, Gardenstyle with Mushrooms & Onions (Ragu)	½ cup	80	0
Spaghetti Sauce, Gardenstyle with Extra Tomatoes, Garlic, & Onions (Ragu)	½ cup	80	0
Spaghetti Sauce, Homestyle Flavored with Meat (Ragu)	½ cup	80	2
Spaghetti Sauce, Meatless, (Aunt Millie's)	½ cup	70	0
Spaghetti Sauce with Mushrooms (Prego)	½ cup	140	0
Spaghetti Sauce with Mushrooms (Ragu)	½ cup	90	2
Spaghetti Sauce, Thick & Zesty, with Meat (Ragu)	½ cup	100	2
Spaghetti Sauce, Thick & Zesty, with Mushrooms (Ragu)	½ cup	110	0

TURKEY

Product	Measure/ Quantity	Calories	Cholesterol (mg)
ROASTERS			
All meat and skin, raw	3½ oz	160	68
All meat and skin, roasted	3½ oz	208	82
All meat only, roasted	3½ oz	170	76
Dark meat and skin, raw	3½ oz	160	72

Product	Measure/ Quantity	Calories	Cholesterol (mg)
TURKEY			
Dark meat and skin, roasted	3½ oz	221	89
Dark meat only, roasted	3½ oz	187	85
Light meat and skin, raw	3½ oz	159	65
Light meat and skin, roasted	3½ oz	197	76
Light meat only, roasted	3½ oz	157	69
PARTS			
Breast, with skin, raw	3½ oz	157	79
Breast, with skin, roasted	3½ oz	189	74
Giblets, simmered	3½ oz	167	418
Leg, with skin, raw	3½ oz	144	70
Leg, with skin, roasted	3½ oz	207	86
Neck, simmered	1 neck	274	186
Skin only, roasted	3½ oz	442	113
Wing, with skin, raw	3½ oz	197	70
Wing, with skin, roasted	3½ oz	229	79
TURKEY PRODUCTS			
Breast, barbecued (Louis Rich)	3½ oz	135	57
Breast, Oven Roasted (Louis Rich)	3½ oz	110	34
Breast, Hickory Smoked (Louis Rich)	3½ oz	125	46
Breast Tenderloins (Louis Rich)	3½ oz	145	36
Canned	3½ oz	163	na
Diced, seasoned	3½ oz	138	na
Drumsticks, Smoked (Louis Rich)	3½ oz	150	82
Ground Turkey (Louis Rich)	3½ oz	225	92
Patties	1 patty	181	na
Wing Drumettes (Louis Rich)	3½ oz	160	80

Product	Measure/ Quantity	Calories	Cholesterol (mg)

VEAL

Note: Figures are for lean and fat unless otherwise noted.

Product	Measure/ Quantity	Calories	Cholesterol (mg)
Arm steak, cooked	3½ oz	298	90
Blade, cooked	3½ oz	276	90
Chuck, braised	3½ oz	235	90
Cutlet, cooked	3½ oz	277	90
Flank, stewed	3½ oz	390	90
Foreshank, stewed	3½ oz	216	90
Loin, broiled	3½ oz	234	90
Loin chop, cooked	3½ oz	421	90
Plate, stewed	3½ oz	303	90
Rib, roasted	3½ oz	269	90

VEGETABLES

Note: All vegetables are cooked unless otherwise specified.

FRESH

Product	Measure/ Quantity	Calories	Cholesterol (mg)
Alfalfa sprouts, raw	3½ oz	41	0
Artichoke	1 large	44	0
Asparagus	½ cup	15	0
Asparagus, raw	3½ oz	22	0
Avocado, California	1 medium	306	0
Avocado, Florida	1 medium	339	0
Bamboo shoots, raw	1 cup	36	0
Beans			
Black-eyed peas	½ cup	86	0
Brown	½ cup	80	0
Butter	½ cup	138	0
Fava	3½ oz	na	0
Lima	½ cup	89	0
Mung	3½ oz	51	0
Pinto	½ cup	78	0
Snap	½ cup	16	0
White	½ cup	79	0

Product	Measure/ Quantity	Calories	Cholesterol (mg)

VEGETABLES

Product	Measure/Quantity	Calories	Cholesterol (mg)
Bean sprouts, raw	½ cup	13	0
Beets	½ cup	33	0
Beets, raw	½ cup	23	0
Beet greens	½ cup	18	0
Broccoli	½ cup	20	0
Broccoli florets	½ cup	20	0
Broccoli, raw	3½ oz	32	0
Brussels sprouts	½ cup	20	0
Brussels sprouts, raw	½ cup	24	0
Burdock	½ cup	123	0
Cabbage			
Chinese	½ cup	8	0
Green	½ cup	10	0
Green, raw	½ cup	12	0
Red, raw	½ cup	16	0
Savoy, raw	½ cup	6	0
Carrot	½ cup	15	0
Carrot, raw	½ cup	15	0
Cauliflower	½ cup	14	0
Cauliflower, raw	½ cup	10	0
Celeriac	3½ oz	36	0
Celery	½ cup	9	0
Celery, raw	½ cup (1 stalk)	8	0
Chard	½ cup	15	0
Chard, raw	3½ oz	25	0
Chiles, red, raw	2 oz	53	0
Collard greens	½ cup	29	0
Corn on the cob	4″ ear	100	0
Corn, sweet	½ cup	65	0
Corn salad, raw	3½ oz	21	0
Cucumber, raw	½ med	8	0
Dandelion greens	½ cup	33	0
Dandelion greens, raw	3½ oz	45	0
Dasheen, raw	1⅓ corms	98	0
Eggplant	½ cup	19	0

Product	Measure/ Quantity	Calories	Cholesterol (mg)
VEGETABLES			
Eggplant, raw	½ cup	16	0
Endive, raw	10 long leaves	10	0
Fennel leaves, raw	3½ oz	28	0
Garden cress, raw	5–8 sprigs	3	0
Ginger root, raw	1 oz	14	0
Indian spinach, raw	3½ oz	19	0
Kale	½ cup	15	0
Kale, raw	½ cup	12	0
Kohlrabi	½ cup	18	0
Leek	3–4 medium	52	0
Lentils	½ cup	96	0
Lettuce			
Butterhead, raw	3½ oz	14	0
Iceberg, raw	3½ oz	13	0
Romaine, raw	3½ oz	18	0
Lotus root, raw	⅔ segment	69	0
Mushrooms, fried	4 med	78	0
Mushrooms, raw	10 small	28	0
Mustard greens	½ cup	31	0
Mustard greens, raw	½ cup	3	0
Okra	8–9 pods	29	0
Okra, raw	½ cup	13	0
Onion	½ cup	29	0
Onion, raw	1 med	38	0
Parsley, raw	10 sprigs	4	0
Parsnips	½ cup	66	0
Parsnips, raw	½ large	64	0
Peas	½ cup	53	0
Peas, raw	½ cup	56	0
Pepper			
Green bell	½ cup	17	0
Green bell, raw	1 large	22	0
Red bell, raw	1 large	22	0

Product	Measure/ Quantity	Calories	Cholesterol (mg)
VEGETABLES			
Potatoes			
French fries (cooked in veg. oil)	½ cup	71	0
New	2 small	18	0
Sweet, baked	1 small	141	0
White, baked	1 med	95	0
White, raw	1 med	76	0
Radishes, raw	½ cup	7	0
Rhubarb, raw	½ cup	15	0
Rutabaga, raw	½ cup	28	0
Scallions, raw	5 med	45	0
Shallots, raw	2 oz	41	0
Sorrel	½ cup	19	0
Spinach	½ cup	26	0
Spinach, raw	1 cup	7	0
Split peas	½ cup	112	0
Squash			
Acorn, baked	½ med	86	0
Butternut, mashed	½ cup	50	0
Hubbard, mashed	½ cup	37	0
Summer	½ cup	8	0
Taro, raw	½ cup	65	0
Tomato			
Green, raw	1 small	24	0
Red, boiled	½ cup	26	0
Red, raw	1 med	33	0
Red, stewed	3½ oz	27	0
Turnip	½ cup	17	0
Turnip, raw	½ cup	20	0
Turnip greens	½ cup	12	0
Watercress, raw	10 sprigs	2	0
Zucchini, raw	½ cup	7	0
CANNED			
Asparagus	½ cup	16	0
Bamboo shoots	1 cup	21	0
Beans			
Baked	½ cup	109	0

Product	Measure/ Quantity	Calories	Cholesterol (mg)

VEGETABLES

Product	Measure/ Quantity	Calories	Cholesterol (mg)
French style	3½ oz	15	0
Italian	½ cup	17	0
Refried, Old El Paso	½ cup	100	0
Snap	½ cup	11	0
Beets, Harvard (Libby)	½ cup	91	0
Beets, Harvard (Stokely Van Camp)	½ cup	80	0
Beets, pickled	½ cup	90	0
Carrots	½ cup	21	0
Chilies, green	2 oz	14	0
Corn	½ cup	50	0
Hominy, white	½ cup	70	0
Hominy, yellow	½ cup	60	0
Mushrooms	½ cup	26	0
Onion	3½ oz	29	0
Peas	½ cup	39	0
Peas and carrots	½ cup	37	0
Pimientos	3 med	27	0
Pumpkin	½ cup	41	0
Sweet potatoes	½ cup	135	0
FROZEN			
Artichoke hearts	½ cup	32	0
Beans			
Bavarian Style (Birds Eye)	½ cup	108	12
French style	½ cup	33	0
Green Beans in Cheese Sauce (Birds Eye)	½ cup	156	3
Italian	½ cup	28	0
Lima (Fordhook)	½ cup	88	0
Snap	½ cup	22	0
Broccoli	½ cup	27	0
Broccoli with Cheese Sauce (Birds Eye)	½ cup	166	4
Broccoli in Hollandaise Sauce (Birds Eye)	½ cup	105	55
Carrots	½ cup	34	0

Product	Measure/ Quantity	Calories	Cholesterol (mg)

VEGETABLES

Product	Measure/ Quantity	Calories	Cholesterol (mg)
Cauliflower	½ cup	20	0
Cauliflower in Cheese Sauce (Birds Eye)	½ cup	162	3
Corn	½ cup	88	0
Corn, Jubilee (Birds Eye)	½ cup	119	1
Corn, sweet	½ cup	88	0
Crowder peas	½ cup	95	0
Kale	½ cup	28	0
Mixed vegetables			
Beans, Cauliflower, & Carrots (Birds Eye)	½ cup	20	0
Beans, Corn, Carrots & Onion (Birds Eye)	½ cup	32	0
Beans, French style with Almonds (Birds Eye)	½ cup	52	0
Beans, French style, with Mushrooms (Birds Eye)	½ cup	29	0
Broccoli with Almonds (Birds Eye)	½ cup	56	0
Broccoli, Cauliflower & Carrots (Birds Eye)	½ cup	27	0
Broccoli, Cauliflower, & Carrots in Cheese Sauce (Birds Eye)	½ cup	128	3
Broccoli, Cauliflower, Corn & Pasta in Parmesan Sauce (Birds Eye)	½ cup	108	2
Broccoli, Cauliflower & Red Peppers (Birds Eye)	½ cup	25	0
Broccoli, Corn & Red Peppers (Birds Eye)	½ cup	49	0

Product	Measure/ Quantity	Calories	Cholesterol (mg)

VEGETABLES

Product	Measure/ Quantity	Calories	Cholesterol (mg)
Broccoli, Green Beans, Onion & Red Peppers (Birds Eye)	½ cup	27	0
Broccoli, Shells, Onions & Mushrooms in Swiss Cheese Sauce (Birds Eye)	½ cup	104	2
Broccoli & Water Chestnuts (Birds Eye)	½ cup	33	0
Brussels Sprouts, Cauliflower, & Carrots (Birds Eye)	½ cup	30	0
Carrots with Brown Sugar Glaze (Birds Eye)	½ cup	82	0
Carrots, Peas, & Onions (Birds Eye)	½ cup	48	0
Cauliflower, Green Beans & Corn (Birds Eye)	½ cup	36	0
Chinese Style Vegetables (Birds Eye)	½ cup	79	Tr
Corn, Green Beans, & Pasta Twists in Sauce (Birds Eye)	½ cup	108	1
Corn & Peppers (Green Giant)	½ cup	86	0
Far Eastern Style Vegetables (Birds Eye)	½ cup	80	Tr
Italian Style Vegetables (Birds Eye)	½ cup	130	0
Japanese Style Vegetables (Birds Eye)	½ cup	98	Tr

Product	Measure/ Quantity	Calories	Cholesterol (mg)
VEGETABLES			
Mexicana Style Vegetables (Birds Eye)	½ cup	125	0
Mixed Vegetables in Onion Sauce (Birds Eye)	½ cup	107	1
New England Style Vegetables (Birds Eye)	½ cup	128	Tr
Peas & carrots	½ cup	49	0
Peas, Carrots, & Onions (Birds Eye)	½ cup	41	0
Peas, Carrots, Pasta, & Onions in Parmesan Sauce (Birds Eye)	½ cup	122	2
Peas & Cauliflower in Cream Sauce (Birds Eye)	½ cup	118	1
Peas and mushrooms	½ cup	73	0
Peas and onions	½ cup	71	0
Peas & Onions in Cheese Sauce (Birds Eye)	½ cup	165	3
Peas & Potatoes in Cream Sauce (Birds Eye)	½ cup	140	1
San Francisco Style Vegetables (Birds Eye)	½ cup	99	Tr
Spinach & Water Chestnuts (Birds Eye)	½ cup	29	0
Stir-Fry, Cantonese Style (Birds Eye)	½ cup	53	0
Stir-Fry, Chinese Style (Birds Eye)	½ cup	31	0
Mustard greens	½ cup	21	0

Product	Measure/ Quantity	Calories	Cholesterol (mg)
VEGETABLES			
Okra, cut	½ cup	26	0
Onion	½ cup	40	0
Onions in Cream Sauce (Birds Eye)	½ cup	105	1
Peas	½ cup	67	0
Peas in Cream Sauce (Birds Eye)	½ cup	136	1
Potatoes			
Hash Browns (Birds Eye)	½ cup	72	0
Hashbrowns (Ore-Ida)	6 oz	130	0
Puff (Birds Eye)	½ cup	192	32
YOGURT			
Apple (Melange)	6 oz	180	6
Breakfast Yogurt, all fruit flavors (Yoplait)	1 cup	230–250	12–19
Banana (Dannon)	1 cup	240	10
Banana, Custard Style (Yoplait)	6 oz	190	10
Blueberry (Dannon)	1 cup	240	10
Blueberry (Dannon Fresh Flavors)	1 cup	200	10
Boysenberry (Dannon)	1 cup	240	10
Cherry (Dannon)	1 cup	240	10
Coffee, lowfat	1 cup	194	11
Coffee (Dannon)	1 cup	200	10
Dutch Apple (Dannon)	1 cup	240	10
Exotic Fruit (Dannon)	1 cup	240	10
Fruit flavors, lowfat	1 cup	231	10
Lemon (Dannon Fresh Flavors)	1 cup	200	10
Mixed Berries (Dannon)	1 cup	240	10
Mixed Berries (Dannon Extra Thick)	4.4 oz	130	10

Product	Measure/ Quantity	Calories	Cholesterol (mg)

YOGURT

Product	Measure/ Quantity	Calories	Cholesterol (mg)
Mixed Berries (Dannon Hearty Nuts & Raisins)	1 cup	260	10
Orchard Fruit (Dannon Hearty Nuts & Raisins)	1 cup	260	10
Peach (Dannon)	1 cup	240	10
Pina Colada (Dannon)	1 cup	240	10
Plain, whole	1 cup	139	29
Plain, lowfat	1 cup	144	14
Plain, Lowfat (Dannon)	1 cup	140	15
Plain, Nonfat (Dannon)	1 cup	110	5
Plain with Honey, Custard Style (Yoplait)	6 oz	160	14
Raspberry (Dannon)	1 cup	240	10
Raspberry (Dannon Extra Smooth)	4.4 oz	130	10
Raspberry (Dannon Fresh Flavors)	1 cup	200	10
Raspberry, Custard Style (Yoplait)	6 oz	190	10
Strawberry (Dannon)	1 cup	240	10
Strawberry (Dannon Extra Smooth)	4.4 oz	130	10
Strawberry (Dannon Fresh Flavors)	1 cup	200	10
Strawberry Banana (Dannon)	1 cup	240	10
Strawberry Banana (Dannon Fresh Flavors)	1 cup	200	10
Vanilla, lowfat	1 cup	194	11
Vanilla (Dannon)	1 cup	200	10
Vanilla (Dannon Hearty Nuts & Raisins)	1 cup	260	10
YOGURT DRINKS (DAN' UP)			
Exotic Fruit	1 cup	190	10
Mixed Berries	1 cup	190	10
Raspberry	1 cup	190	10
Strawberry	1 cup	190	10
Strawberry Banana	1 cup	190	10